ONE STEP AT A TIME

ONE STEP AT A TIME

Francesca Giacomozzi

Cherish
EDITIONS

First published in Great Britain 2021 by Cherish Editions

Cherish Editions is a trading style of Shaw Callaghan Ltd &
Shaw Callaghan 23 USA, INC.
The Foundation Centre
Navigation House, 48 Millgate, Newark
Nottinghamshire NG24 4TS UK
www.triggerhub.org

British Library Cataloguing in Publication Data
A CIP catalogue record for this book is available upon request from
the British Library
ISBN: 978-1-913615-23-9
This book is also available in the following eBook formats:
ePUB: 978-1-913615-24-6

Cover design by BookCollective
Typeset by Lapiz Digital Services

To the souls who are tired of living a life dictated by their mental health: may this book help you realize how worthy you are of living a full, satisfying, loving life.

My long-winded journey into a fuller and healthier self. Written with the hope that if you are lost, you will soon be found. This is the honest and unfiltered truth about me and my experiences as a warrior in eating disorder recovery. All the people mentioned in this book are real, and therefore have been made anonymous unless they provided consent to be spoken about by name.

ABOUT THE AUTHOR

Francesca Giacomozzi has lived in the UK since April 2016.

After quitting a full-time job that wasn't fulfilling her, she studied to become a yoga teacher and reflexologist and now owns her own yoga teaching and massage therapy business.

Her drive to help others overcome mental health issues has pushed her out of her comfort zone, leading her to raise awareness about eating disorders as a daily mission.

Francesca has two degrees and can speak five languages.

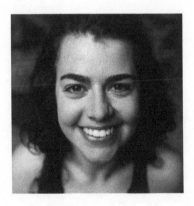

ABOUT THE AUTHOR

CONTENTS

SEA WISDOM

I sat by the sea
And I observed the water breaths
Flowing in and out of me

I couldn't get my head round
How strong and powerful something so liquid could be

And then one day it hit
Tiny drops of shifts
That's what the ocean is.
Waves teach us
That nothing
Ever lasts in its original form
Waves teach us to cope
With the swings of the ocean
Sometimes
Being afloat
Isn't quite enough.
When a storm hits,
You have to dive deep
Into the unknown
To be able to come up
Through the other side.

STUDLAND:
THE TIPPING POINT

06 August 2016

Dear diary,

Fran here. Curly-haired, quite loud, and very optimistic chick.

Today, I'm setting off to walk the South West Coast Path, a 360-mile footpath that runs across three counties in England: Dorset, Devon and Cornwall. It is the UK's longest and most loved national trail, and it starts (or finishes) just outside my doorstep.

Well, that isn't quite true. It's not *my* doorstep. I moved to Bournemouth a couple of months ago to refresh my English and take a bit of a break from my Italian life. I worked as a school matron at Bournemouth Collegiate School, but now that it's summer I've ended up staying at my stepdad's friend's house. Random, I know, but I needed somewhere to crash and they needed a house-and-dog-sitter, so it worked out well.

On my long evening walks with the dog in Poole Park, I kept observing the land that appears on the horizon: Old Harry Rocks and the whole peninsula of Studland. I'd heard amazing things about that side of Dorset, and slowly a plan to undertake a solo excursion manifested itself. I wanted to break free and dive into the wildest nature I could find around here – chipping away at everything that had been weighing me down.

Even if I consider myself to be a little bit of a lone wolf, this will be the very first time that I have set off on an adventure of this kind. It will be a raw, slow journey, just me, myself and I. Well, actually, me, myself and my backpack. My beloved bright green 35-litre Vaude Brenta, in which I have managed to pack away everything I will need for the two-week walk.

I have learned from thirteen years of Scouting experience that the less I pack, and the more compactly, the better my physical and mental experience will be. I'm not quite sure if people who have never belonged to such groups will understand the powerful lessons the Scout Association teaches. Yes, maybe people make fun of us because we walk in shorts in the winter and carry big rucksacks up mountains. However, there have always been those 'Eureka' moments in my trips away with the Scouts that have left me loving nature like it is a part of my body (and appreciating little luxuries like running water and a gas hob). Most importantly, though, there is this feeling of leaving something heavy behind. Just as our bags become lighter and lighter the longer we walk, as we eat our food supplies, the lighter our souls become when we realize we need only our legs and lungs to hike up a mountain and overcome obstacles – both mental and physical – along the way.

Yes. It's as simple as that. Which is perhaps why I'm so convinced this trip can save me.

***

It feels so weird when you get up and the only thing that reminds you that you are alive is the big mirror in the hall on the way to the bathroom. I stare at the image reflected in it every damn day. I analyse every single imperfection, every single edge, every single spot. I've tried so many times to avoid that reflection. It really bothers me. I wish I didn't have to see my big fat arse, my face full of spots. I am certain nobody else wants to see it either. In the past, I tried to fake it and pretend to be happy. I tried to cover my sadness and insecurities by eating the entire contents of my fridge, by going out in the evening, partying hard, drinking until I forgot who I was, smoking my head off... but doing none of these things changed the fact that, actually, I felt like shit. I felt so shit that my bad days started to become my new normal, and my good days turned into a distant memory.

Well, here we go, then. No mirrors, no make-up, no fancy dresses – nothing but my hiking boots and a couple of comfortable T-shirts. Just a path to follow and my headphones, in case I get tired of my own thoughts (which happens quite a lot). Sounds perfect.

As I approach the beginning of the coastal path, I get a stunning view of Old Harry Rocks, which makes me more and more excited about my hike. If the sun shines and my eyes can capture scenery like this, I think I can go quite far.

All I had to do was jump on a bus and get a ferry across the peninsula, and now I am walking through a nudist beach. The guidebook I purchased before the walk had actually warned of the potential scenes of bums and genitals, but what surprised me most was that the beach was full of elderly people, living their most relaxed and shameless lives right there in front of my eyes. I am very intrigued by this concept of older people not giving a damn about social decency, but I also need to avoid staring at them in case they think I am a weird pervert.

I feel like I am walking on clouds, and there is a gentle breeze caressing my smile. I am encountering so many different people along my way, but because I am approaching the path in reverse, starting from the end of the recommended guidebook route, there is not a soul walking with me; everybody is walking toward me. I calculate that there are roughly three minutes between the time that people first spot me and shout a greeting to the point where I'm too far away to hear them. In this short window of time everyone asks me questions about my life, my origins, my plan for the walk. At first it is fun and nice to chat with strangers, but then it becomes like a repetitive and not-so-pleasant nursery rhyme:

'Where are you off to?'
'Penzance, ideally.'
'Where are you from?'
'From Italy.'
'Are you on your own?'
'Yep!'
'Enjoy your walk then – and be safe!'

I guess maybe they are not used to seeing a girl with a big backpack hiking at the speed of light (at least, that is how fast it feels to me), but I wish I could just record my answers and play them back from my phone when needed.

***

It gets quite annoying when the only thing that people ask about you is where you are from. I feel like they are intrigued more by my accent than anything else I could tell them about myself. I say I am from Italy and they immediately brighten, as if they have just encountered a cute little exotic animal in the wild. 'Hey, mamma mia!' some will say.

I wonder what it is about being from Italy that people find so fascinating. I have been Italian all my life, but I have never understood what's so special about it. It's just a country. Borders and nations are so arbitrary, in my opinion, that I sometimes really struggle to see any difference at all among my fellow humans. I would much rather say I'm from Earth or something.

I am not even sure I fully belong to Italian ground. I feel so out of place in my home town. Which is probably why I have been dreaming of a life outside of Italy ever since I was 16, in the hopes that travel would alleviate the heaviness I was feeling in my heart.

I'd heard a Scout friend talking about the opportunity to spend a school year abroad, and then next thing I know I'd signed up to spend ten months in Germany. The hardest part was convincing my parents that it would be a good idea. The second hardest was deciding whether I was going to leave my boyfriend, or try a long-distance relationship.

All I knew was that I couldn't wait to leave my life behind. I felt so stuck, and figured the only way out was to physically get away.

***

Twenty-three miles later, my feet are so sore that I can barely take them out of my hiking boots. I have covered so much land today; I went from Poole Harbour all the way to Kimmeridge Bay, passing through groups of people picnicking on the path or abseiling down the cliffs. My eyes have seen so much beauty, only ruined by the volume of plastic left behind by uncaring visitors. I am happy I made it to this bay just in time to watch the sun set. I sit quietly as I cook my dinner on the stove, trying to override the voices in my head that are whispering to me to skip dinner, so that I'll certainly lose weight. This is my very first night, and I am wild camping in a bivvy bag generously donated by E.T., one of the only two guys I've hung out with since I moved to Bournemouth.

I am telling myself not to panic, but what looked like an amazing place at sunset, has quickly turned into a very scary place in the dark. Better focus on finding the best spot to place my bivvy bag. That way, I might not even notice I am all alone in the middle of nowhere. And eventually, there will be light again!

***

I had never been a fan of the dark, until I realized it is the best time of day for me to hide all of the things I don't want to see anymore. Like my own body. Or these thoughts that make my head spin. Some days, I wish my whole life away into darkness. A silent, numb and infinite dark space where I can float, emotionless, in peace. My body is a burden and I want to fix it, but how do you fix something that doesn't hurt physically? Some days, I am in so much pain that I want to hurt myself to give other people real reasons to look after me. Maybe if I break a leg, I will get all of the attention I need. I might even get help for my head. I see no other way out at the moment.

***

I look down at my feet and I get shivers from the state of my blisters. How am I supposed to walk all the way to Penzance with these feet now? It's only day one, and I am already half ready to go home. What if they start bleeding? What if I can't get back anymore? What if people see I am vulnerable and try to attack me? I want to go home already. I am such a failure. I hate this body so much, I want to throw it in the bin and get a replacement. I literally cannot even see one project to completion. I might as well just go back to the only thing I clearly do so well: eating until I am so full that I forget who I am.

Luckily, my overthinking process gets interrupted as I'm spotted by a couple in a caravan parked a little higher up the bay, who offer me a cup of tea.

'There is no need to thank us. A cup of tea is just boiled water.'

'Still. That is lovely.'

'So, are you on holiday?'

'Well, I guess it still feels like a holiday, but I've moved to the UK for good.'

'Have you?!'

I respond with my customary wide smile.

***

My eyes sometimes betray my smile. It's been kind of a crap year for me. I had to go through a lot of stuff, and I'm not over it yet. But at least I am aware of it, I guess. Sometime before this trip I purchased you, diary, where I thought I could keep track of the amazing experiences I was having while living in the UK, but what I wrote instead was this:

Hi, I'm Fran and I've got a binge-eating disorder (that's what Google says, at least). Food is both my best friend and my worst enemy. Love and hate. It allows me to survive, but it also kills me. I spend almost all of my time on this earth literally obsessing over what I want to eat and what I have to do in order not to gain weight.

I hate people who are able to eat whatever they want, whenever they want. I hate myself because I work my arse off to lose weight and then I always screw it up when I binge.

I hate myself for doing it, but I hate myself most for being too weak to stop. I hate myself even for hating myself! I can't love myself. I do not like my body or my skin, and I especially hate my arse. Way too big. All my friends back home have better bodies than I do, and I'm really jealous, to the point that I stopped getting ready and dressing up for the evening with them.

I binge, and I feel so ashamed of doing it. It scares me to think that people might be able to see me bingeing, so I usually wait until I'm alone. I crawl out at night, when no one is around, to eat all the things that I kept away from during the day for fear of being judged. I also pay a lot of attention to what other people are eating and I normally try to calculate the calories of every single meal, theirs as well as my own.

I am obsessed with food because it gives me unconditional pleasure. I don't have to ask for it; I can just get it from the fridge or purchase it from the supermarket. I sometimes force myself to eat to the point where I just swallow everything I can find until I feel sick and am unable to move.

And when I reach that point, I start to feel guilty for what I've done to myself, and I'm filled with self-loathing for having ruined every effort I'd been making to eat better and be healthier.

I tell myself, people are starving in the world, and you are eating until you are not only full, but to the point you feel so sick that you can barely move, you disgusting monster.

I didn't even know this was a real issue until I decided to research my behaviours and feelings on the internet. That was when I discovered more facts and information about binge eating and yet, even if I can now name the demon that resides in me, it still scares the crap out of me.

***

'Are you okay?' the caravan couple ask me.

I must have gone silent for a while.

'Yes,' I reply, 'thank you. I'm just a little tired. I might go back to my bivvy bag, but thanks for the tea. I appreciate it.'

ASHES

Hey I found this picture the other day
I wonder
If you actually stayed
Like I promised you I would
But then I started feeling the wounds
Of the weight on my shoulders
Life it ain't calmer
The world is not a better place
And I thought having you far apart
Would mean I could depart
From the thoughts of being yours
Of having us
Turns out,
what I refused to be once
Doesn't scare me no more
Is there a chance
I can walk back through that door?
The days are tough out here
They left me with no fear
Of what will be of my relentlessly hopeless wandering
Excuse me again you know
I was just wondering
How low
You think of me and everything we
Saw
Cause I still feel

We could see
A brighter light
Something small but fine
Something uplifting
From the sorrows of the past and
The worries of the last
time I saw you.
Hey I found a picture the other day
Too bad,
It was just a flame.

JURASSIC COAST:
NOTHING IS THE SAME ANYMORE

07 August 2016

I wake up from my first night wild camping to a drizzling sky at 6am. I am the only one within at least a two-mile radius. There aren't even any campervans.

I decide to seek cover under the roof of the public toilets, so at least I can pack properly without getting wet. And then off I go toward Lulworth Cove. I would love to reach Weymouth, but I am afraid my blisters will not let me. I never thought my beloved hiking boots – which walked with me for kilometres and kilometres of Dolomites and Apennine paths – would let me down so badly on the first day of this adventure.

Note to self: do not attempt ten hours of walking on the first day. But how could I stop feeding my eyes with such beauty? The scenery was so stunning, I just couldn't get enough. Like with food. But better. Because hiking doesn't make you fat, right?

Anyway, I feel like crap today. The weather is grim: I can't see anything apart from my feet squelching away on a muddy hilly track, and one thought keeps going round and round in my head: why the hell did I decide to hike on my own? I knew that I would lose motivation at the very first rough patch. And now, the only thing I can do is keep walking, even though my feet are killing me and I am still completely exhausted from yesterday. If only I could see the sea today. It would definitely help distract me from this hard walk.

Six miles – seeming to be the longest six miles of my life – separate me from Lulworth Cove. I can make it. Well, I have to!

***

I've been to Lulworth Cove once before. It was the day I was heading back to Poole after spending five days at Camp Bestival, where I volunteered for eight hours to get free access to four days of pure festival madness. I was tired, covered in mud, and very stinky, but definitely feeling way better than when I'd arrived. I had just been sacked from my summer job and I was feeling absolutely useless. It's not that I enjoyed being a waitress, but it was either that or go back home to live at my mum's for the summer. And for some reason, I didn't want to go home. Maybe it was mostly because I didn't want them to find out about my eating disorder. And maybe because I didn't want them to think I was going crazy.

Luckily, my host family suggested I apply for work at the festival. I ended up having an amazing time and meeting a few people I will never forget.

C is one of them. C and I shared so many details of our lives, it almost felt like we were twins who'd been separated at birth. We spotted one another as we were pitching our tents in the same camping spot. Two minutes into the conversation in English and we both realize we're Italians. It wasn't only the coincidence of finding another connational at a random British festival, but I also discovered we studied the same course at uni and we were born only three days apart from one another. I immediately felt such a strong connection with her. One night, I confessed to her things that I had never told anyone about; things that I was still really ashamed of.

I told her about my ex and how I ended the six-year-long relationship with him on Skype. When we met I was 14 and he was 13. I saw him for the first time in one of those mixed tournaments we used to do with the Scouts, and I immediately had a huge crush on him. Like, real bad. I couldn't take my eyes off him. He was athletic, spontaneous and a little mysterious. He was also gorgeous, but I only cared about that smile, and I soon realized I just had to get to know him.

Fast forward a couple of years, and after an incredible number of MSN chats and a few dates gone wrong, we are together. This time we are both really into it, so it was too bad that, just a few weeks later, I had decided to leave home and go to Germany. I was in a very confused state. I loved him so much, and I was convinced we would be together forever if we managed to survive ten months apart. And so we did. We were strong: we stayed together despite everyone's opinions, and that to me was the ultimate proof that true love existed, and I didn't need anything but him. But there was something at home that was suffocating me, and I needed to escape, so I kept going away. Then, when he left for study reasons and I stayed at home, we didn't last. Or, rather, I didn't last. If I had the power to travel back in time and do one thing, it would be to give my tipsy, needy self a slap, and stop me from cheating on him. I had never done anything so disrespectful and hurtful to anyone in my life, but it happened and I couldn't reverse it. It was something that was going to stay with me forever and I had to face the consequences of my actions. I tried to tell C that it was almost like I felt this urge to fuck things up because I was feeling stuck, to untie all the strings that were attaching me to this person, even though I knew I was going to be lost without him. I told her I felt disgusting and so unworthy of anyone's respect that I wanted to disappear from this earth. That my pain was truly deserved because if I was capable of hurting the only person who I thought I truly and deeply loved, then I must be a heartless monster who deserved nothing but the worst in life.

C just looked at me with compassionate eyes, put a hand on my shoulder and told me that everything was going to be just fine.

And just like that, for the first time in a very long time, someone had listened to my story without judging me for my actions, without giving me their opinion on the most painful and embarrassing experience of my life. For the very first time in a long and painful year, I had finally been listened to, and this simple act of kindness from her made my sorrows feel slightly less heavy and somewhat more bearable to carry. I definitely thank the universe for bringing us together, as she really made me feel like I was less of the monster I'd conjured up in my mind.

***

I'd better check where I am. Three miles to go. How can that even be possible? I've been walking for almost three hours today, which means I've only done one mile per hour. Does that mean I am going to be stuck here in the wet weather for the night?

With this heavy fog, I have no indication that I am still on the right path and the only reference points I have are from my guidebook. I know that to my right there are a number of military training ranges used by the Armoured Fighting Vehicles Gunnery School and to my left, sheer cliffs. Perfect day to get lost. In any other situation getting lost would just mean that I need to find my way back to the right track, but in this situation, getting lost means either falling down a cliff or potentially getting run over or shot by the military.

I want to cry. Actually, I'm already tearing up. This always happens whenever I try to achieve something; I underestimate the challenge, push too hard, expect everything to go the way I want it to go, and then I don't have the strength to suck it up when things don't. I am so mad at myself right now. What an awful idea this was. The South West Coast Path will be the end of me.

'Are you alright?'

Out of the fog, two figures walking their dogs on the path near the cove cautiously approach me, obviously concerned about my welfare. While I struggle to contain my tired tears, their beautiful dogs are ironically having the time of their lives, as they disappear from my sight and into the fog, running, jumping and wagging their tails. These two figures, two middle-aged men who are now standing right in front of me, also don't seem particularly bothered about the misty, gloomy weather, and the way they speak to me is very calming and it makes me feel safe.

'Hmm, yes?'

'You don't really look happy.'

'Oh, well, I'm just a bit tired I guess – my feet are killing me.'

'Did you want to give us your backpack for a while?'

'Thank you, I'm okay ... but maybe you could keep me company?'

'Yeah, can do. So, are you here on holiday?'

'No, I moved here. For good! Five months ago almost.'

'Oh wow, what brought you here?'

'Hmm, well, my stepdad is British. He was born in Poole and moved to Italy more than 30 years ago. He met my mum six years ago and they got together. Basically, I've swapped lives with him. He is living where I was born, and I am living where he was born.'

'How random!'

'Yeah, I mean, I thought it could be a good chance to settle down in the UK before I start my master's degree. Although, I'm moving up north.'

'Whereabouts?'

'Manchester.'

'Oh, you're gonna miss this place! The north is cold and grey.'

Great. Now *that* comment is definitely going to make my life easier. The only thing I am sure about right now is that I want to start uni again, and hopefully this time find a career that I enjoy. And now these two fellas who I don't even know are making me doubt my choice of location, the only decision I was certain about.

Sometimes people talk without a filter, and that's okay. I wish, however, my mind was tough enough to learn how to sift through the passing comments and opinions of other people, but I simply can't do that yet. Instead, they drag me down a rabbit hole of insecurities and over-reflection, where the only thing I feel is lost.

We walk for more than an hour before we reach Lulworth Cove, and believe me, I am trying so hard not to appear really happy to see so many people around me again, but I bet I look like a castaway, impatient to touch firm ground as we approach the coffee shops and restaurants.

The last time I was here, I remember looking across the cove and admiring its almost perfect semicircular shape and the bright blue reflection of the water. Nonetheless, this time round all my eyes can see is a grey strip of sand and a crowded car park. I must be looking really desperate, because the lovely rescuers invite me to have a late breakfast with them at one of the cafés. I accept the invite, quite surprised by how casual and natural this whole situation feels. I give their dogs a good cuddle while I munch my way through the first warm meal I've had in two days.

***

Isn't it impressive how meeting caring people can become the moment you show up for yourself and ask for help? I think the tiredness and desperation of finding myself in uncharted waters knocked the pride out of me. I don't think I would have asked for help on any other occasion, but I did then, and I am very grateful for it. I am safe, I feel better and I have a full belly.

I don't understand why we're so determined to succeed by ourselves all the time. It is almost a deadly sin, asking for help. And then, when we do find the courage to, it's really hard to trust anyone. We feel bad about telling people that we don't feel mentally okay, because we are worried they are going to think less of us for it. We are conditioned to think that showing some vulnerability will just put ourselves in a dangerous position, when the real danger is not allowing our emotions to ever surface. We're told to toughen up as if being stoic and thick is the only way to survive. But if our struggles were physical, we wouldn't think twice about asking for a hand, nor would we feel like we are such a burden to other people. I am tired of hiding behind physical symptoms to get the attention that I deserve for my mental health. I am tired of pretending that I will be okay on my own, when I know all I need is a little help.

***

As I thank my new friends over and over for their kindness, the fog begins to lift, leaving space for a mild temperature and a blue sky. They call it the 'Great British Summer' but I think that the 'Great British Scam' is a little more appropriate for these sudden shifts in the weather. I try to take a deep breath and decide to focus on my next move. Durdle Door, a stunning and incredibly famous natural arch made of limestone, is just one mile away, but I can't walk it – my feet are swollen and soaking wet. I enquire with the local hostels about room prices and availability for spending the night in Lulworth Cove, but, as expected, the prices are insane. I simply cannot afford to spend that much money on only my third day of what will be a two-week-long trip.

There are only two options remaining: either take the bus or hitchhike to Weymouth. Both choices mean I will have to miss out on going to Durdle Door, but I know that if I go, I will have to spend the night outdoors there, and I really don't want to do that.

Luckily for me, after a good hour of unsuccessful hitchhiking attempts, and just as I am about to give up and buy a bus ticket, I manage to catch the attention of D, a surfing instructor who is returning home after running his outdoor sessions. He stops after seeing my thumb sticking up and offers me a lift to Weymouth. I step into the van, feeling cared for and I fill D in on my plans for the rest of the trip.

'Nice to meet you, D, and thank you very much for the lift again! That was really nice of you.'

'Good luck for the rest of your walk, Fran.'

'Thank you! It will be a long way but I am ready!' I reply knowing that what I am saying is a lie. Fake it until you make it, right?

I step out of the car, in socks. I have taken my hiking boots off and my feet are beginning to feel alive again. I look around with curious eyes, taking in all the details of my new home for the night. As I waddle barefoot toward the seafront, I get the impression that Weymouth is the classic place for family vacations. There are big terraced houses, all lined up to face the promenade, and an abundance of ice-cream kiosks and fish and chips stalls. I inhale the salty sea air and feel the warm sand beneath my feet.

I decide to sit somewhere and soak up what's left of the sun to try to feel a little less cold. I am pondering whether to buy myself an ice cream (everyone I see seems to be enjoying one), but just the idea of it brings a lot of unwanted thoughts in my head: how much I am going to regret it, how much sugar and fat an ice cream contains, how much more walking I will have to do to burn those calories off and how fat I already look and therefore don't deserve it. I wish I could make all of these feelings disappear, but it only happens when I feel loved and cared for.

***

I wish receiving love and affection from people was as direct and effortless as eating food. I just have to open my mouth, grab a bite and feel the flavours comforting my palate. Chocolate is my new way of hugging; bread is my way of finding strength.

I don't remember when I first started finding comfort in food. It kind of took control over me gradually, and then before I knew it I was just always suffocating my feelings with food. I slowly lost control of my own actions, lost control of my own mind and now the worst thing is that I have no one to talk to. I am alone here, having to go through it all by myself. I left the only person I used to talk to about my moods. He was the only one able to absorb my thoughts and help me feel better about myself. Now look at me; I can't even bloody decide whether to get an ice cream or not because I keep hearing the same three sentences in my mind:

I gained weight.

I am unworthy of love.

I should definitely disappear.

***

The sun is melting my thoughts into an exhausting, self-destructive process and I'm just so overwhelmed by it. I look ahead and I see perfect little waves of salty water calling my name. Being in water, feeling fresh and clean is very appealing right now, and I would love to have this as my last memory of the day, rather than my everlasting stream of horrible thoughts. However, that means conquering the social anxiety that comes with undressing. I take a deep breath, and as I do I look around me to see if anyone is looking my way.

I slowly undress to the sun, still seated, letting go of some of the layers of clothes I am wearing, and then quickly, super self-conscious about having my big, short legs and my belly fat exposed, I head into the water, where I can hide my disgusting body again from any unwanted looks.

***

Every summer, I dream of having a 'bikini body'. I even purchased a book called The Bikini Body Guide. It states that I will be able to get the perfect body shape to wear a bikini and simply feel comfortable in it. Finally, all of those social occasions I missed out on for fear of being too fat and too ugly, I will be able to attend!

All of the meals I said no to, I will be able to eat! All of the clothes I haven't worn, I will be able to wear comfortably without having to hide parts of my body away. Yet, every single summer, I am continuously disappointed, because, once again I have failed to get fit.

I think it is unfair how beauty is unevenly distributed – that some people seem to have perfect genes and others, like me, seemingly drew the short straw. I hate that I am so weak mentally that I can't stick to a training routine and meal plan like every other woman on this earth seems to be able to do. How can I be loved if I am not beautiful? How can I attract people I like if I do not feel attractive? But, most importantly, how the hell will they love me if I can't even love me? My mum keeps reminding me of this. 'You need to love yourself, darling,' she says. But I honestly do not understand how to do that without getting physically fit first.

I feel like I am losing my grip on everything I once thought was certain. I can't think of one single thing in my life that is the same as it was a year ago. It has been the worst year of my life so far. I am weak and needy and my mood depends almost completely on external appreciation – especially boys'. I have started doing this thing now where I have to have a boy in my bed because, otherwise, I can't sleep. But then, even after I've got all of the things I thought I wanted from them, I still feel worthless and empty. Yet I continue to do it, again and again. Part of my brain tells me this time will be different, this time I will encounter 'the one', but it never is, and I never do.

Maybe I have left 'the one' behind me and will never find anyone like him again. I feel so much pain, but I don't even know if I'm entitled to feel it, because I did this to myself after all. I wanted this relationship so much and then I burnt it to the ground. My first love. My sun, my home, my compass. He was all of these things and more. But I broke up with him and now I am alone.

I honestly think I am literally the worst person in the world. I feel so lonely it hurts. I keep longing for someone to arrive and *show me the way out, carry me out of here, rescue me. I have no idea why, but I feel so incomplete on my own. I sometimes feel as if I am missing an arm or a leg without him. Despite the pain of missing this metaphorical limb, I need to trust that this time I was given on my own is the time necessary for me to grow my own leg or arm. And as much as I know that I need to feel good alone, I still have absolutely no clue how to do that. Like zero idea. On top of that, I keep having these massive doubts about whether the time for meeting a person who shares my interests and complements my personality is over already. Whether, while I was having a long-term, long-distance relationship, I missed out on everyone being single, and now that I'm single, everyone else has decided to jump onto the relationship bandwagon.*

Is it true? Is this a real thing, or is it just my anxiety talking?

***

'You alright?'

A ginger boy with sleeve tattoos and a cute smile is talking to me from across the beach, I must have been staring at him while I was thinking of my ex. Great.

'Oh, well, I am, but I need to find a good camping spot for the night because there are no vacancies whatsoever... Do you know a place I can camp at?'

'I'm sorry, no idea, but, I mean, I know it might sound dodgy, but if you're desperate, I can host you. My place is really small, but I would never let anyone sleep on the road.'

Again, someone else offering help! It must be my lucky day.

I decide not to take up this stranger's offer right away, but to keep the option available. I head back toward the promenade, feeling the need to be surrounded by people. While I sit on a bench, I lose myself looking at the blue sky and watching seagulls feeding themselves off leftovers near the chippy.

I contemplate the simplicity of life – such as moments passing and never returning, waves creating and then destroying themselves – and I wonder if there is even any sense in all of this? In humankind, I mean. We convince ourselves we are here on this earth for a reason, but is it really this way? Or are we just one of the many evolutionary coincidences happening on this planet? If the latter were true, then why do we delve so much into our past, and future? If all we are is a random act of creation, then our meaning here on this earth has nothing to do with our past nor future and a lot to do with how we decide to live each moment for its presence.

After around ten very unsuccessful enquiries at some local B&B and hostels, I decide to take the ginger boy up on his offer, and head for his house. At least I will not be alone with my own thoughts this evening, and I can eat hot food, and potentially even have a real shower. Really I just need some comfort and some human company.

GROWING UP

No one ever said
It was going to be hard

No one ever said
that taking up more space
Was going to hurt

Growing tall
Whilst
Rooting down
At the same time

Growing up is a stretching process
Expanding limits
Of the body
And the mind

Growing up
Is a harsh task

The skin and its stretch marks
That's how I feel inside as well

And every time
Growing doesn't come easy

I feel like
I'm ripping apart

And I want to quit
And stop hurting
Choose comfort
Over growth
Choose safe
Over challenging
But then I remember

Butterflies break free
 from their past lives
Before they can fly

CHESIL BEACH:
I AM SO LOST

08 August 2016

'Thanks, S. It was nice of you to host me, and thanks for offering pizza last night.'

I am packing at the speed of light because it was a very weird night. I appreciated his hospitality, but I did not know he had such a small apartment and I ended up having to choose between sharing the bed with him or sleeping on a very dirty floor. I went for the second option. I thought I was going to enjoy my stay at S's house but it turned out he'd basically just invited me over because he wanted to have sex with me and it felt really uncomfortable. I was able to say NO and move his hands away from my body, but I am lucky he listened to me. It could have gone so much worse.

***

This encounter has left me with some seriously mixed feelings, but I guess it was my choice to put myself in the home of a random person, right? I should have been more aware of the fact that the situation was uneven in power, that I am a girl travelling on my own and he is a man offering me a place to spend the night.

I really hate all of this guilty fear that is pervading my soul. I feel like a horrible human being just for saying yes to free accommodation, because I should have known better... I should have remembered my mum's warnings of all the terrible things that can happen to a girl when she is on her own. What is appropriate to wear and what isn't. Which situations are controversial and potentially dangerous, and which type of guys we should trust and which we shouldn't.

Quite frankly, however, I am tired of living in fear. Just because I was given these genitals instead of others doesn't give anyone a valid excuse to invite themselves in. I am tired of being constantly afraid of the opposite sex's apparently 'uncontrollable instincts' that make them hunt girls as if they were fresh game. And this world is doing a great job, justifying rapes and sexual assaults as little boys' pranks – 'boys will be boys' after all. Why do we always downplay the responsibilities and actions of sexual predators and blame the survivors? Do they not go through enough as it is? You can find lists and lists of things that we, as women, shouldn't do, but, not once have I heard of a list of actions that men should avoid taking in the first place. Why is the world so upside down?

***

I leave pounding through town, following the signs for the South West Coast Path that are positioned throughout Weymouth for hikers like me. I decide to focus my energy and anger on the goal of the day: Abbotsbury. I have just checked in the guidebook, and it says I need to head over to Portland Beach Road in order for me to find the coastal path. The sun is still out, shining bright, and I feel okay, all things considered. I take a deep breath and I tell myself that life goes on, and so does my journey along the South West Coast Path.

'Hey, sir, excuse me! Do you know where Portland Beach Road is?'

'Yes, that's in the same direction I'm heading toward now. Do you want a lift?'

I am not sure how exactly, after the night I had, I still trust people, but this gentleman seems genuine. And I am exhausted from living in fear of constantly being attacked just because I am a woman. So I take a chance and jump into the back seat of his car.

I feel grateful because, as it turns out, J from Yorkshire had been planning to go diving, but because of the uncertain weather he was now going to a triangular shaped peninsula named Portland instead. He drops me off right between Weymouth and Portland, on the tiny strip of land that connects the two.

All I see ahead of me is a little wooden bridge and a horizon of sand and sea. I am so psyched again to walk and devour land with my feet; I cannot wait. Without hesitation, I start walking along the coast, following Chesil Beach. To infinity and beyond! I feel, once again, as if I'm in one of those movies where the protagonist starts strong and finishes even stronger, where the soundtrack is so upbeat and motivational and the highlights of the quest are incredible and she is so light with her steps it looks like she's almost levitating toward her destination. Sounds too good to be true, right? Well, actually, yes.

Three, four miles in, panting and struggling to move forward, I begin to wonder why my progress feels so slow today. I look ahead of me at what I thought was a compact path, and I realize with a sinking feeling that it has just been a continuation of the pebble beach all along. I have been making progress in the way of two steps forward and one step back. The sweat is dripping down my neck and I already feel dehydrated, so I check my guidebook: 'Chesil Beach is an 18-mile-long shingle barrier beach stretching from West Bay to Portland and is considered to be one of Dorset's most iconic artificial landmarks. The coastal path detaches from it at the very beginning to leave space for a little lagoon that separates the two.'

I realize with terror that I have set off on the wrong side of the coastal path.

After a few grunts and swearwords, I accept my fate as I stare at other hikers in the distance, across the speckle of water, walking graciously on soft ground: I am lost, again. In fact, lost isn't really the right word for the situation I now find myself in. I know where I am, I am not lost. I am just in the wrong place, and not only am I in the wrong place, I have taken the path of absolute pain and desperation.

***

It's ironic. This is a very accurate exemplification of how I feel mentally. I know now that there is only one way for me to end this long journey of pain, and that is to push through, to get to the end of it. Because while turning back is an option for this physical journey, it certainly isn't for what I am going through in my head. Fuck. I don't know if I can do it, in all honesty. I am scared that I won't make it on my own but for some reason I also don't want to bother my loved ones, because I feel really stupid.

I hoped that a geographical reset might help, that maybe being away from home would help me rediscover my definition of self, like a brand-new start, away from all the expectations I felt growing up. Yet,even now that I have removed myself from the environments that I thought were no good for my wellbeing, I am still struggling to understand who I am.

All of the things that used to make me me, all of the 'titles' I used to describe myself with, like being a girlfriend, a student, a Scout, are all gone and I don't know who Fran is anymore. The only thing I know is that I can't afford to lose this battle. I know the only way out of this turbulent time is to get to the bottom of these feelings. I need to figure this out, or I know I'm going to end up hurting myself physically because I can't bear my mental pain anymore.

***

God, it's hot out here. So hot that I am concerned that this little trip is not going to end well for me at all. I am starting to worry about becoming dehydrated. I tell myself it is time to stop for lunch: a can of tuna and some oat crackers. I am glad I prepared packs of emergency food. I guess wearing ridiculous uniforms and singing Christian songs around the campfire weren't the only things that stayed with me after 13 years of Scouts.

Aside from worrying that I won't make it, I only have two options: keep going until this shingly hell reunites with the rest of the land, or turn back and start again on the right path. The idea of retracing all those painful steps really couldn't sound any less appealing, so I reluctantly decide to keep my head down and just keep moving forward.

I had decided to only use my phone for emergency situations, but this feels like it's getting perilously close to being one, so I take my headphones out and blast 'Hopeless Wanderer' by Mumford & Sons on repeat, which seems rather fitting for my current situation and will at least give me some light relief from my relentless mind chatter.

Four hours and forty-three minutes later, – not that I am counting – after hearing the same lyrics over and over, and singing from the bottom of my lungs to the most beautiful song ever written, I believe I am seeing a mirage. I spot a humanly figure right in the centre of the speckle of water between beach and land, rowing a boat. I start running like crazy, waving my arms in the air trying to attract this person's attention. Once again, I feel as if I'm auditioning for *Castaway*.

'Hey, Hi! Hi, Hey!'

This indistinct blob that looks like a miniature person waves at me and then keeps rowing away. *Shit!* I run even faster. This time, the blob starts becoming more man-shaped, and then finally I can hear his deep voice. Out of breath, I explain my predicament.

'Sorry to bother you... but... I'm lost. I don't know how I managed this, but I ended up walking on Chesil Beach instead of the marked South West Coast Path.'

I introduce myself and he does the same, and as he catches the desperation and tiredness running through my eyes, he offers me a lift across the lagoon. He has two beautiful dogs with him and they wag their tails at me and give me a few licks on my very dirty and sunburnt hands once I'm safely on board.

I am so thankful I bumped into him, but even more thankful that he appears to be quite an introvert. I am totally wiped out, and there's no way I could even try to express what a journey it has been so far. I stare at the water to try to avoid eye contact, because this man looks far too much like my grandpa.

***

I miss you, Nonno. I miss you so much. I hadn't realized how special you were until you left this earth. I can't believe I didn't get a chance to say goodbye to the man who raised me to be a strong, curious and independent woman. I still remember the day I came to your hospital bed and you held my hand and told me you loved me. You also thought I was Grandma for a little bit, which was quite funny.

I also remember that I promised you I would see you again. That that time wasn't going to be the last time. But it was. I left for China and you left for good. The illness you had was a tough one for all of us in the family; we could see your light growing weaker and weaker each day, your attentive and curious eyes becoming more and more lost, searching for some long-faded memories of all the people around you.

I wish I had thanked you for all of the incredible times we had together before those memories vanished from your head. I love you and miss you dearly. One day, I promise I will make you proud. I will raise children with good values and work ethics like you taught me.

***

'Listen, Little Miss Lost, I am heading home. Do you want me to give you a lift to Abbotsbury? You can meet my wife, maybe have a cuppa, and there's also a bus stop just outside my house. You can take it from there if you want?'

In all honesty, I feel like this walking adventure is starting to become more of a hitchhiking adventure, and I don't know whether I like the sound of it. I mean, let's face it, people will hear about my two-week hike and then they will ask me how much effective walking I've done. Ha. What can I say? Maybe I won't tell this story to anyone. But yes, dear G, I would very much like a lift, so I can get as far away as possible from this hell on earth.

I end up having a nice chat with him and his wife, a good cuddle with his beautiful dogs, and a cup of warm tea while wrapped in a blanket. What a treat! They talk to me briefly about their children and a lot more about the history of Abbotsbury.

When I get to the bus stop, I decide to sit on the bench and try to recap my options. Luckily, this town's bus connections are so limited, it is basically a no-brainer. Bridport lies in the centre of all the public transport connections here in Dorset, so it's clearly the best direction I can head in right now in order for me to stay on track.

The bus arrives, saving me from a classic 'Great British Summer' change of weather. What was once a sunny, warm and welcoming day has suddenly become miserable, with heavy rain and thunder and lightning. I sit in a corner of the bus and put my headphones in, hoping to go unnoticed. I am too exhausted for small talk. Before I delve deep into my internal world, I notice a few people on the bus wearing fancy dresses and glittered hair.

***

I love festivals; they are the perfect environment for me to get rid of all the layers of insecurity and just let go, exploding with joy and fun. I dance to the music of the different stages until there is nothing left in me. The rhythm, the music, the lights, they all combine in the perfect cathartic release for my emotions.

It is why I also used to dream of becoming a professional dancer. When I was 16, I was really close to auditioning for bursaries and trying to take the big leap. I remember putting music together to create the hip-hop remix to which I would have performed. Lights on stage, I would express all of these super heavy and burdening emotions that were flowing constantly through my body, so that I could make people witness my internal struggles. And hopefully this would be cathartic enough for me to finally be at ease with myself.

I used to close my eyes and imagine myself performing at the finals of Just Debout, an international hip-hop dance competition. Too bad I never had the courage to actually put myself in front of a judge. I was scared of being told I was too fat to dance competitively, like I was told by other ballet teachers years before. I think my fear of failure outweighed my fear of missing out on the opportunity, but I remember a time when my guts weren't always wrenching and twisting in a knot, when my head wasn't always wrapped up in the anxiety of what's next.

I remember I used to have vivid dreams and hopes for the future, where I'd see myself as an incredible traveller, and mother and partner, too. But now all of it seems to have vanished into a very intricate maze of choices. Where have my dreams gone?

There was a time when I could see nothing between me and my goals. And now? I end up craving food instead of emotions. Physical fullness instead of mental fullness. No matter how hard I try to fill myself up, all I feel is numbness and emptiness. I really want to find that spark, that impulse, again. I need something that keeps me alive. Literally. I also think this might be the key to healing all of my wounds: having a purpose again – having something to hold on to that will allow me to reverse the self-destructive path I've mistakenly taken.

***

As we slow down, I realize I have been in my head for so long that we have nearly reached Bridport. I look out through the window and notice the bus is coasting downhill through the highstreet and a girl, who is striding purposefully on the pavement next to the bus, catches my eye. She has beautiful ash blonde hair and a confident attitude, and for some reason she inspires in me a sense of tranquillity. The bus makes a sudden turn down a smaller and bumpier road, and it comes to a stop, as I lose sight of her. Everyone seems to be getting off, so I assume we have arrived at the bus station.

SOME DAYS MORE THAN OTHERS

I can withstand
The knot of uncertainty
insecurities
Fears
Dissatisfaction

Some days more than others
All of it together
On my skin, in my guts
I suffer
The ebb and flow
Strong and deceiving

Some days more than others
I can grip the ground
Resist
Survive
Breathe
Observe

Some days more than others.

LYME REGIS (PART ONE): THE RIGHT SUPPORT

Staring at the bus routes poster, in a foreign country, while receiving a lot of unwanted attention (I do look slightly homeless at this point), it is not the easiest setting for me to make a concrete decision on where I want to go next. After a couple of episodes of acute social anxiety, I am trying to just put one foot in front of the other and make small decisions.

My mind is playing ping pong between two opposite ideas: keep being a hero (knowing for sure that I will not make it to Cornwall), or get on the bus, allow my ego to die a little, and admit it was a pretty crazy idea from the start to think I could walk for 300 miles in two weeks with little to no training. I am also aware that I need to stay as close as possible to the coast if I want to arrive in Penzance within my deadline.

***

I don't know why, but I feel guilty jumping on another bus. I feel like the experience of leaving my comfort zone and hiking 300 miles on my feet is my only chance to heal from this misery and addiction that I have. I am scared that allowing myself to rest properly won't actually have an impact on how I really feel about myself.

Ugh, if only I had prepared myself better for this. If only I had slowed down on the first day, if only I had planned the route better... IF ONLY will certainly become my nickname if I don't stop overthinking everything that happens to me.

I wonder if my mind regretting and rethinking past actions has to do with the unrealistic belief that we need to be good all the time in order to be considered a good person. As if even making one little single mistake might take us straight to hell, ruin our reputation and put shame on our family name. I only realized how rooted 'being perfect' is in our upbringing when I started considering myself a failure every time I was not making the 'right' choice. What even is a right choice, anyway?

Every time I decided I wanted to think, say, wear or feel something different than what it is considered to be normal, I found myself being judged, misunderstood, bullied back to the only path that our society accepts. The quest for perfection. I knew there was something wrong with it, but I didn't truly 'get it' until I felt it weighing me down. I started comparing myself to the unnatural beauty standards of television and magazines. I started wishing I didn't have body hair, skin flaws, belly rolls. I picked apart my entire physique and found something wrong with most parts, and then did the same with my clothes, my hobbies, my relationships. It all had to fall into the 'aiming for perfection' category and I stopped allowing myself to make silly mistakes, be adventurous and explorative with my own life because of this ridiculous standard people are asked to uphold every single day of their life.

At this point, I am starting to question all of my beliefs because they only seem to be doing me harm and no good. So I think that, for today, it is okay for me to just be human and get on a goddamn bus.

***

I eventually get on a bus toward Lyme Regis, the closest destination that is still on the coastal path that I can reach from Bridport. To my surprise, I notice that the girl I saw earlier has got on too, and she is heading to my favourite seat. Upper deck, front seat: the spot where you feel like every single turn in the road is too sharp to make, and every tree branch is going to crash into the window and leave you beheaded.

Apparently, I make this comment out loud without realizing and she returns my attention, asking about my hiking boots. She seems really impressed by my idea of walking on my own on this path and so she keeps asking for details of the journey. After the classic get-to-know-the-stranger conversation, Rebecca, that's her name, wants to know where home is for me and where I am heading.

Good questions. Superficially, easily answered. But in depth, I don't think I know the answer.

***

Only a traveller will understand the beautiful agony of feeling like you belong in all the places you've been to, yet, at the same time, feeling at home in none of them. Not long after I left Italy, I discovered that there is a point of no return, when you realize that your concept of 'home' has changed forever.

While before, 'home' was a distinctive place on earth, made up of a single geographical location, at some point after I spent prolonged amounts of time abroad, it started melding into this very transient mix of different cuisines, languages, people, places and feelings. Everything that I was curiously contemplating with my big naïve eyes was slowly permeating my skin to become a part of me forever.

And that is both a blessing and a curse. A blessing, because I was privileged enough to be able to find myself at home in several countries and study or volunteer in beautiful places across the ocean, experiencing first hand and embracing the culture of my host countries. The memories that are connected to each country keep my heart warm and make me proud of my adaptability. A curse, because to feel entirely at home is to feel reunited with all of those places and pieces left around the world at once, which, as far as I know, is impossible to physically do. So, my heart aches often, longing for the unrealistic moment when I will feel at home again. I guess for now, my home is my backpack. And my hiking boots. And all of the memories that live inside my head.

***

'My family is from Italy. I'm heading to Penzance and I will be camping tonight. One of my strongest skills is improvisation, so I will probably end up staying in a park or a field just off the main road.'

'Not a chance. Lyme Regis is very busy in summer; it will be hard for you to find a good place to sleep. I have a spare room and you are staying at mine.'

To my great surprise, she doesn't seem to accept no for an answer, so my wild camping and hiking adventure has just turned even more than before into a hitch-hiking and hospitality-seeking trip. She is adamant that one more person in her house will not make much difference. Becca lives there with her boyfriend and her best friend. The bus stop isn't far at all from her house and I get a warm welcome from everybody there when we arrive. She shows me the guest room, and as I take my shoes off, she points out that my feet look terrible and my blisters will need time to heal before I even think about walking any further.

I slowly start to give in to the idea that I may have to stay here for a night or two. We start sharing stories about who we are and I end up telling her I speak five and a quarter languages, and that I'm learning to rock climb. I ask her about her life too. Becca is a cook; she enjoys slow cooking and local ingredients.

She loves feeding people. And I hate feeding myself.

Great combo, right?

***

I always try to avoid tasty meals because I feel like they might make me crave even more food than usual. I aim for bland choices so that I can stop eating it because I don't enjoy it. When I go to the supermarket I spend hours and hours checking the labels for the number of calories contained in each food and I am always researching which foods will take me more calories to digest than the calories I am consuming from eating them in the first place. I obsess with how many carbs I eat in my meals because during my time researching countless diets, they all unanimously say to cut carbs down. I also stopped going out for lunches and dinners where possible because it makes me very uncomfortable, eating in public. I never want to be the person who gets their meal first because I don't like to see the people around me eating when I have already finished. It makes me want to jump onto their plate and help them polish off anything they have left.

Everywhere I travel there are a lot of restaurants that do buffets and they are the worst possible scenario for me, as I am faced with a bottomless pit of food I can't choose from, and I just end up eating everything until I am so full I can't even walk or breathe properly. I also tried to imitate the girls in the movies, where they make themselves sick after eating, but I am such a failure that I can't even do that.

This impulsive eating makes me feel like an animal. I am so ashamed of myself.

***

I feel the need to explain myself to Becca so that she won't judge me too much if I have one of my binge-eating attacks, and I try to approach this incredibly difficult conversation that I've never had with anyone before. I am a little reluctant to open up to a stranger, but for some reason, perhaps because in all probability I will never see her again, I don't feel awkward. As I tell her, not a word comes out of her mouth. Instead, she simply listens to me, with her big blue Irish eyes wide open, and the moment I start to get a little upset she gives me a huge, suffocating hug.

All I will remember from today will be this: I spoke about my inner demons for the first time to another person and they didn't think I was a monster. Sometimes all you need is someone to listen instead of giving you advice.

CRAVING THE LIGHT

I keep longing
For a ridiculous
Amount of clarity

I forget sometimes
Clouds hold more meaningful sights
Then an empty sky

Serenity doesn't necessarily mean
I'm awake
And connected

Fog and grey
could be triggering
Rain
Life
Growth
Light

LYME REGIS (PART TWO):
MAYBE THERE IS A WAY OUT

09 August 2016

I wake up feeling rested after a good night's sleep in the cutest guest room I could possibly wish for, and I notice I feel weirdly lighter today.

***

I think vocalizing my battle helped ease my nerves a little. I have been scared all this time to give a voice to the vast darkness that lives inside my mind for no reason. Maybe talking about it isn't so bad after all. Becca definitely didn't seem shocked or alienated by the things I told her. It was as if I had simply said, 'You know, I've fallen off a bike once, and it hurt.' She almost dealt with this huge burden of mine as if she had been through it herself.

Even though I am grateful, because opening up made things a little easier in my mind, at the same time I am raging because I wish I could have had this conversation with my parents or at school, instead of talking to a stranger whom I just met.

Why did I only find out at the age of 23 that eating disorders include an actual complex series of mental health struggles related to food? All I heard about was anorexia and even then I was told that only life-threatening anorexia was a real issue, as if only the illnesses that you can see with your own eyes are real. Why do we give so much attention to our physical health, yet learn nothing about mental health? Where is the mental health awareness week in schools? How do parents forget to mention to their children that their health is not just the sum of their physical characteristics but it is actually also how they feel on the inside?

***

I spend the day flip-flopping around the beautifully curated gardens of Lyme Regis, alternating between soaking up the sun and hiding in the shade of some large trees as I read a book and write my thoughts away. As I return to the house, Rebecca announces excitedly we are having freshly caught fish for dinner and we will grill it on a portable BBQ on the beach. Becca, her boyfriend and her best friend are making me feel so welcome that I almost forget we've only just met. We are all sitting on the promenade, laughing our bellies off, partly because we all are a little bit tipsy from the copious amount of beers we've drunk but mainly because it is ridiculously windy and we are barely managing to hold down all our things from blowing away.

Before dusk, Becca makes a joke about my horrible blistery feet and suggests I should stay until I feel ready to go. I am speechless. I don't know how to say yes without making it look like I am taking advantage of them, but I'm really enjoying their company – and I *do* have horrible blisters… Also, I have heard the coastal path gets tougher from here onwards until Cornwall, so I figure I'd better stop trying to be a hero and allow myself to rest and heal properly before I attempt the second leg of the hike. I'm only human after all.

At breakfast on the third day of staying with Becca, I realize this is the first time in years I have enjoyed a tasty coffee and croissant without feeling terrible about it afterwards. This gives me some strength, and I decide to take some time today to try to figure out when exactly my eating disorder started. I need to go back to the beginning. The very beginning.

***

It feels incredibly hard to travel back in time and pinpoint the exact moment I started having a terrible relationship with food. I think it partially stemmed from the obsessive television-watching I did when I was in my teens. My parents were working a lot, so not having much more company than my grandparents and MTV, I definitely spent a lot of time growing up watching skinny girls shaking their booties to rappers and boy bands.

On top of that, my whole family often used to compliment my looks rather than my mind, so I guess that is also a big reason why I over-identify with my physical self. When all you hear for over 20 years of your life is how 'pretty', 'gorgeous' and 'beautiful' you are, it's no wonder you start to believe you need to be all of those things to be worthy of attention and love.

I think the worst was when my grandma would feed me enough food for three people and then comment on how big my bum looked. Or when she would tell me how thin she was when she got married. They may seem like trivial comments, but when you're a girl blossoming into your teenage years, having to deal with all of the internal changes that puberty brings is hard enough without the extra focus on how you look or people pointing out that your face is spotty or that you need to be below a UK size 8, otherwise you're fat. And then, as soon as you hit 16, all of the diet talks you have always heard around Christmas, New Year, just before summer or any other vacation, begin to insinuate in your mind. Your worth is equal to your weight on the scale you keep checking every damn day.

***

'Hey, Fran, what was it you said the other day, about going to Brazil?'

'Yes, my travelling career – as I like to call it – started when I was 17 and I left home for the first time on my own to study abroad. I wanted to go to the States but my parents were terrified about sending me to the other side of the world, so I settled for Germany. Little did I know, I still had to attend school and take A-level classes if I wanted to pass and get into the final year of college.'

'Right... but how does that relate to Brazil?'

'Oh, that's where I met AA. He was from Brazil, he was a year above me in school, and was doing the exchange in Germany as well. He told me all about his country and it sounded amazing, and so, a year later –after finishing all of my A Levels and college, and waiting for university entrance exams to open – I decided to go and volunteer in a Christian community in Brazil for three months.'

'Wow, that's crazy.'

***

The craziest part of this trip was that I nearly ended up taking the vows. I was so close to just calling my family and telling everyone I was going to stay. I was searching so hard for my own meaning and I honestly was so lost after college that I did not know what I wanted to be in life. All of my childhood, I thought that finishing compulsory school would have been enough to know who I was going to become. However, I realized that I had focused so much on the finish line, that I forgot to figure out who I actually wanted to be. I had no idea whatsoever what I wanted to do with my time, my knowledge. So when I got to Brazil and was given a new mission and an objective, I thought I found my purpose. Giving my whole self to a higher cause has always been my dream, but I never really considered the consequences of doing so. I prayed with the nuns every day for a sign from God or the Universe to show me my way but I am still here, four years later, without a calling, without a reason to be alive.

***

'Oh my God. You climb, you hike alone, you speak all these languages, and you've lived in five countries. Who are you, an MI5-trained spy? So unsuspicious but yet, with all these mad skills?'

Becca cracks me up with her comments. This makes me laugh, not least because I consider myself the clumsiest person on the face of the earth, and a special agent wouldn't have gotten themselves lost twice in two days either. We spend the evening pub-crawling, chatting, eating and drinking together, and I feel joy pervading my soul for the first time in a very long time. Sadly, these feelings of joy and affection are short-lived and a sense of restlessness kicks in at the exact moment I realize that I am leaving tomorrow. I feel the same nauseous yet excited feeling I get when I am about to leave a beautiful chapter of my life to move on to the next one. I stare into the night sky wondering if this is all there is – the constant changes and my incessant need to move and shift, pushing and pulling my destiny to try to make the most of my time on this earth.

I go to bed with this mind chatter every night and I wake up feeling insecure of anything and everything about my life. I am just hoping the wine will calm my mood and help me sleep. Tomorrow is a big day and I really need to rest.

***

I remember I always struggled sleeping as a kid. Especially when my mum would work night shifts and I would be taken to spend the night at my dad's house or at my grandparents'. I don't remember what would trigger my anxiety, but I clearly remember falling asleep in front of the telly next to my dad, and then all of sudden being told to go to bed. And the moment that would happen, I would for some reason be instantly wide awake again. Worrying about having to go to school the next day. Worrying whether I had done enough homework not to be caught unprepared in a surprise exam (there are a lot of these in Italy). Worrying about the fact that if I didn't stop worrying, I wouldn't be able to sleep and wouldn't be rested.

I had so many of these episodes that my dad would really struggle to put me to sleep. I would try to resist the temptation of getting in the bed between him and his partner, and then after what felt like three hours of terror, I would be walking in the dark, crying, toward my dad's bedroom door. At first, he would try to help me sleep by coming to read me a fairy tale or something. But then it didn't go away, and I think he thought it better to give me some tough love instead. That didn't work either, and this anxiety stayed with me until I was around 12 or 13.

I really don't think I've ever overcome it fully because now I feel the exact same sensations as I did when I was a kid I would never have imagined that, at 23, I would still have trouble sleeping.

I feel as if there is so much darkness in me, like a huge void that I can't fill. And then there is the raw, indescribable pain that I get when I try to sit with myself. It roars inside me, and I am scared to face it. I am scared to the point that I may hurt myself just to stop these voices, this insomnia, this anxiety of facing one day after the other.

***

10 August 2016

I wake up in the morning to the sound of my alarm. With reluctance and a hint of excitement, I do a body scan and notice my legs feel rested and my feet have healed. There is also something in my body telling me it is time to move on. So, I eat breakfast with Becca and then I jam-pack the very few clothes and my bivvy bag into my rucksack by squashing everything down with my foot and standing on it. I am very much over the packing/unpacking dance I have to do every time I stop in a different place for the night. However, I am still craving adventure, movement, speed.

With a great deal of melancholy, I salute these amazing people who have been my entire family and support for these past few days. I am so grateful; I really hope we can keep in touch. I promise them I will head back for some surfing with them soon. As I close the door behind me, I realize, looking at the main road and a hoard of people descending down to the beach, that Lyme Regis is way busier than usual.

It is time to set off to find the coastal path that I have been observing from the seaside these past few evenings. For once, I actually had a look at the guidebook before I launched myself into another Chesil Beach disaster. Still, I am slightly dreading this Devon trek, which is meant to be as magnificent as it is brutal. The drastic drop of the golden cliffs on the horizon are unravelling into intricate ups and downs and twists and turns, and I am ridiculously underprepared.

***

I think that's it. It's the fear of the unknown, of being unprepared, that makes me cling so much to everything and anyone I can find. That's why I feel so needy. So desperate to find a guidebook for making it through life. For someone to tell me what to do with myself to feel better.

With the increasing awareness of my needs, something else is slowly seeping through, and that is the realization that no one knows what to do, how to act, what to choose.

A lot of the people I have met during this hiking adventure have shared their stories with me, and what I have come to realize is that no two lives are the same. Even when I have heard of people struggling with some very similar issues to each other, everyone has found their own way of dealing with those issues. S was coping with a tough family situation, Becca's friend had faced some disordered eating in the past, and the more I opened up about my own struggles, the more I discovered everyone is also dealing – or has had to deal – with some internal struggles of their own. It was such a revelation to me – coming from a town of closed minded people, where no one speaks about mental health – to actually hear other fellow humans speak their minds.

There is so much pain in this world in general, but I always feel like I'm carrying it all on my own shoulders. When I feel misery in my heart, when I feel broken, it is very difficult to navigate and distinguish between my own pain and that of the world. It is so important for me to be able to separate the two, because the first I can barely work with, while the second is just too much for me; I need to share the load. These conversations I started to entertain have all made me feel less alone, and they opened my eyes to two mighty realizations. Number one, I am not the only one struggling. They may be facing different struggles, but there are a lot of people out there in this world who aren't feeling great either and yet they manage to survive and get through it.

Number two, there isn't unfortunately a one-size-fits-all solution to these issues… and that's scary. It doesn't help me feel positive about my future, because it is clear now that even if I do get help, I won't just find a magical cure for all of my pain. But on the other hand, it gives me a small nudge as to where I need to look in order to find myself again, and to stop feeling so bad about my life. Every person is their own individual self before they identify with a role. Every person has a home before they even understand where they live and that is their own self. I was a person before I was my ex's girlfriend, before I was a

Scout, before I was a student. I had a place that has always been home and always will be, no matter how much I travel or how often I move.

That place is me, my own head, my own thoughts. I believed for such a long time that I had to fix my body or change it before I could feel at ease in it, but I realize now it is my mindset toward my body I need to change.

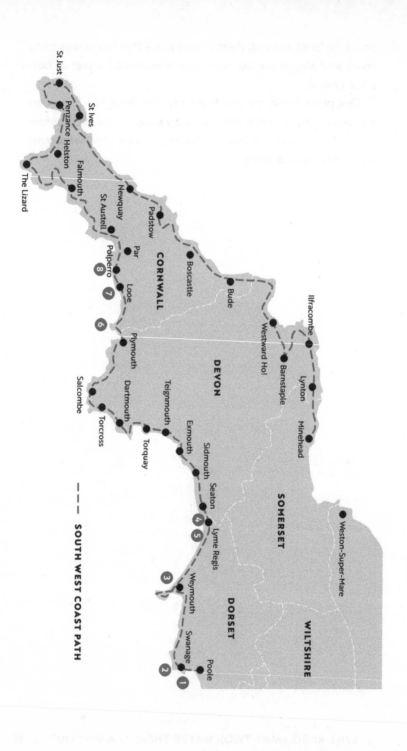

SOUTH WEST COAST PATH

St Just
St Ives
Penzance Helston
The Lizard
Falmouth
Newquay
St Austell
Padstow
Par
Polperro
Looe
Boscastle
Bude
Westward Ho!
Ilfracombe
Lynton
Barnstaple
Minehead
Weston-Super-Mare
Plymouth
Salcombe
Dartmouth
Teignmouth
Torcross
Torquay
Exmouth
Sidmouth
Seaton
Lyme Regis
Weymouth
Swanage
Poole

CORNWALL
DEVON
SOMERSET
DORSET
WILTSHIRE

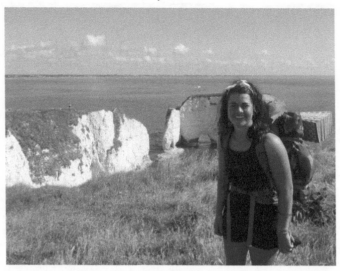

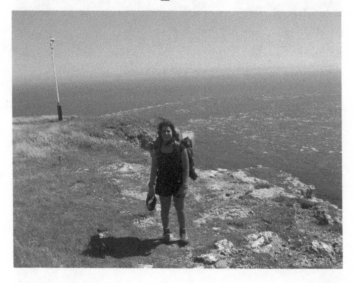

3

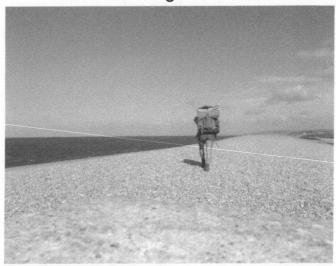

4

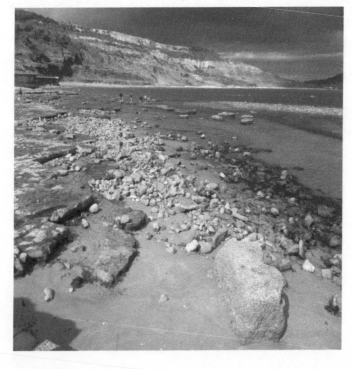

5

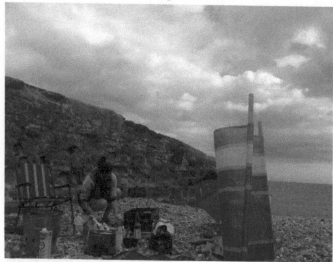

6

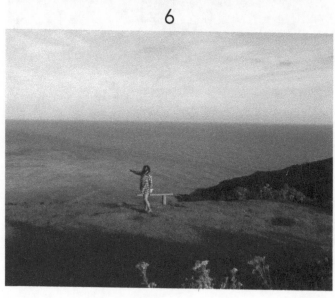

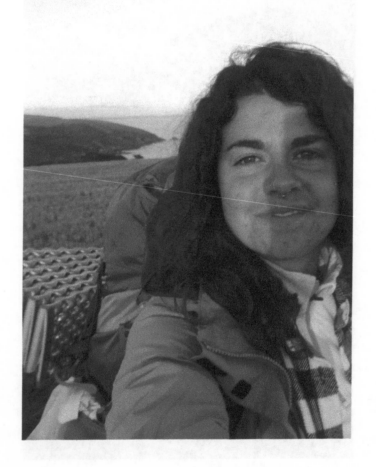

8

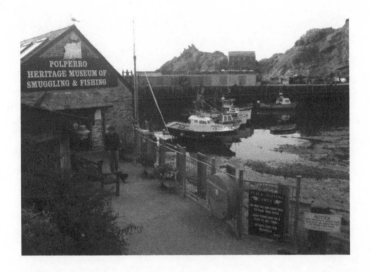

8

WHEN ONLY I CAN

Hello.
Can you tell me
How do you feel?
Not the I'm alright
It's all good
Not bad thanks
kinda interaction,
avoiding conversation
Seeking for inaction
World's a scary place I know
But hiding behind fake words
Is that helping your soul?
Are you choosing numbness over fear?
Cheap thrills over lasting smiles?

I'm guilty too,
For sure

It's easier pointing the finger
Than changing myself

Letting other people be in charge of how I should feel

Letting them handle my fate
As if I didn't have a choice to act
differently

Begging externalities
To give me answers only
I know

Asking other people to be my roots
When only
I can grip ground.

CREMYLL AND POLPERRO:
I AM NOT A FAILURE

The instant I decide to catch another bus to skip the Devon part of the coastal path, I feel weirdly proud of myself. Instead of hating myself for not accomplishing what I set out for, I actually feel okay because I understand my limits now more than I ever did; I firmly believe at this precise moment that there is nothing worse for me to do than not listen to my gut.

I want to have a fairly relaxing trip to Plymouth, so I catch one of those fast buses with air-con and comfier seats. My guidebook says the trail from Plymouth to Polperro is one of the nicest stretches of the whole South West Coast Path, so I am very curious to go and explore by foot. Yes – by foot! No more buses.

As I arrive at my destination, I feel calm but Plymouth is a pretty big city, the first one I've seen in days. I start feeling a little anxious about being surrounded by so many people buzzing around, all knowing where they're heading to, while I, as per usual, feel like I'm struggling to understand which way's up and which way's down. As the guidebook is written for people who are taking the coastal path from Cornwall to Dorset, and I'm doing the route in reverse, I pause for a moment to figure out which direction is best for me to take; I need to find the Cremyll Ferry to take me across the river Tamar. I have absolutely no idea where I'm supposed to get this ferry from, but I assume that it will be near the main ferry harbour. However, when I arrive at the harbour, all I can see are countless oversized ferries, not the one I need.

I can't really say I'm tired, because in reality I've been slacking off on the walking side of this adventure, but honestly even just making decisions and sticking to them feels incredibly hard right now. I'm surprised I've not ended up running in a circle trying to bite my own tail. I try to take a deeper breath in and continue my hunt for this goddamn ferry.

After I have taken a couple of wrong turns and barely managed to avoid a military base camp, I finally find the right dock. I stare out to the sea, waiting for the ferry to approach land. I am amused by how clear the water and the sky are looking today. I had no idea England could ever be so warm and sunny.

I adore the fact that I seem to be the only one getting the ferry, which makes me feel kind of exclusive. I take a lot of pride in thinking I might be the first one doing something. Too bad I wasn't born in olden times, since nowadays almost everything is already invested in, patented, discovered or done. We are just improving, changing, shifting and transitioning from what's already known.

When the ferry starts approaching, I suddenly realize it's a teeny tiny boat. Nevertheless, I proceed to step onto the vessel that will lead me to the beginning of the Cornish trail. As I look up, I see a very attractive guy looking my way. I stare at him for a little longer than necessary and then realize he's smiling at me.

I feel a little flustered. I'm not going to lie – I've been feeling pretty gross since I started the walk, and on top of that, it has been quite a long time since someone I fancied also seemed to be genuinely interested in me. I don't really want to start a conversation this time though, because I am on a mission. The day is already halfway gone, and I really can't fall for another stranger. My self-esteem is crushed already; I don't need another delusional love story.

In what feels like no time at all, my good intentions are swept away by his persistent smile and I suddenly find myself smiling back. Within a few minutes, I am telling him all about my crazy adventure and what I was aiming to do with my time here on the coast.

***

It is remarkable how people seek travels and adventures to get lost and find themselves again. But even more incredible is that people still choose, most of the time, to stick with the person that they know they are, even when they introduce themselves to strangers.

Why do we do that? Logically, if I wanted to get rid of my persona – as in the person that I have always been: my name, my habits, my passions, my feelings – I would think that at the first opportunity I would just start over, make up a new name, a new story. Maybe even a new nationality.

It makes me laugh that even now, when I can't even face my own reflection in the mirror each morning, I still choose to introduce myself to this boy, Toby, with my real name, my real identity, my real hopes and dreams. I choose to be me. Fran. Bubbly, chatty, loud Fran.

This makes me think that maybe we don't go travelling to break away from ourselves as a whole, but from the parts of ourselves that we do not like. Because those are the parts that make us feel unaccepted, rejected. Our shadows are what we fear people will judge. Our demons make us feel embarrassed about ourselves, so we constantly try to hide them.

Despite that, when I opened up to C, and then to Becca, I didn't feel as if my shadows changed their opinion of me. And even now that I'm talking to Toby about everything I can think of, I feel very at ease, as if all of the judgement has been lifted away and any topic of conversation is allowed.

***

We chat for what I believe is a good hour before I come back down to earth and realize it will be dusk soon and I haven't even left Cremyll yet. I have no clue where I will be staying tonight. I try to explain my situation to Toby and I find myself being given a plan of action: ' Go there, walk up to here, wait there, get picked up, stay at mine, continue to walk tomorrow, then maybe I'll drop you off at Portwrinkle, which is a little closer to Polperro.'

I am feeling speechless and also a little annoyed at myself for letting my brain get distracted by my hormones, but I cannot help but say yes. And to be honest, sleeping somewhere inside where there is a soft surface I can lay my head on is way better than bivvy-bagging it in the elements. This might mean that tomorrow I'll need to make up for the time I've lost by reverting to being a teenager again for a few hours today, but there is some sort of light-heartedness that really pulls me in. I feel very at ease and comfortable with this fella I just met, maybe even more so because I find out he has a girlfriend and I know his intentions are not malicious.

'Okay then, Toby, I'll see you at Rame Head!'

Would you trust a stranger telling you to meet him at a cliff point called Rame Head? In any other circumstances I would have hesitated, potentially declined but I have been taking a lot of chances this trip and I feel so alive, for the first time in months, if not years! The walk up from the ferry to Rame Head is the most amazing trek I have ever done. It is hilly, has got loads of ridges, beautiful clear water in the distance, and a dusky sky on the horizon. The best, however, is yet to come, as I arrive at the top of the cliff and discover with a soaring heart that I can see, past the roaring sea, most of the coastline of both Devon and Cornwall so clearly that I feel so in awe of this planet.

As I take in the spectacular view I can feel the tingling sensations in my fingertips and toe-tips again. I can breathe fresh air into my anxiety-crushed chest; I can smell enthusiasm and the wind of change. This is probably the first time, in what feels like my entire adulthood, that I don't feel the need to eat until I'm hurting, because I don't need food to make me feel something. I am having an amazing evening, and finally I can allow my thoughts to stop and leave me here. Dragging one bit of life in at a time. When Toby arrives at the meeting point in his 4x4, we spend a few minutes observing the landscape, telling each other adventure stories and taking pictures of Rame Head.

The night ends with me going to bed with a light heart and a bit of a crush. I almost wish that this moment would never end, but I cheer myself when I realize that it didn't actually take much at all for me to feel okay today.

***

Panta Rei. Everything flows forever. Nothing is ever going to be the same again. A philosophical concept I learned in school and that would always make me feel incredibly anxious about the future. Almost as if, up until now, I thought that my role on this earth was to grip and hold and fight for time to stop and for nothing to ever have to change.

I always felt this incredible urge to fix everything that wasn't working anymore. Even when the price of repairing was more than just letting it go and finding something newer and better.

Except now, slowly, I am coming to terms with it. I now realize the only certainty we can hold on to, is that everything will change. That a sense of joy can be found in leaving the past behind. There is also a kind of happiness in knowing that every step forward means a step away from the things I want to leave behind. Every mile covered, both physically and metaphorically, I am shaping a newer version of me, leaving pieces of myself behind.

***

11 August 2016

Toby drops me off in the morning and leaves me in a huge field full of sheep poop and tall grass. There is a humidity in the air that makes me think I am likely to get rained on soon, so I pull my waterproof jacket out of my backpack. Although, actually, come to think of it, I'm not really that bothered about the weather anymore; it doesn't scare me the same way as it did at the beginning of this adventure.

***

As I observe the silhouettes of the ferns that surround the trail path, I start to wonder why nature always seems to make me feel better. It has been the strongest medicine against all sorts of sorrows in my life. When I am in nature, I feel gratitude for all the times I managed to get myself back on track and dragged myself out of something that wasn't right for me. So hopefully, this time, I will be able to drag myself out of this hole too. Nature teaches me constantly with its beauty that all that matters is enjoying the present moment. Enjoying the natural magic that surrounds me every day, every minute, every second. When rather than walking face-down, or looking at my phone, I start to lift my head up and truly experience the life that surrounds me, that is when I become alive and truly connected with the rest of the world.

***

While immersed in my thoughts, I notice the trail starts descending into a bay. I look frantically at the map and pray that it's Polperro.

Not quite. But the good news is I'm not that far away from it. I can already smell the Cornish pasty and coffee I'm going to have for lunch.

***

Eating. What a difficult topic. It's been so difficult to just think of food as a source of energy. It feels like I'm having a binge attack every time I need to eat.

I call them attacks because I honestly couldn't describe them any other way. When I have one, I almost feel like my body is under siege from an external, very powerful source that commands me to eat until all I feel is full. Then I come back to my healthier self and the realization of what I have done and how much food I've stuffed down my throat and it makes me feel horrible. Unworthy of even trying to find a solution, because I know this will never stop. And just like that, I am once again under siege.

But I need some food, I think, and I am sure I have lost some weight on this walk, so I deserve it.

And there it is. I've done it again. Told myself I deserved food because I lost weight. As if I wouldn't be allowed to eat anything at all if I was fat.

Eating is a biological need, so why is food considered a treat and not a necessity? Why do we associate it with comfort, happiness, relief? Why do I always think that I need to reach the point of starvation before I can eat something? And why am I so obsessed with my body? Surely all I should want is for my body to simply function normally. Instead, I constantly analyse the way I look, the way I pose, the way I stand, the way I talk.

I know this self-destructive mind chatter isn't coming from me, though, not really. It's not something I taught myself. I look at my environment, my world, and I see with horror that we are subjected to this stuff from a very early age. As a society, we are totally fixated on appearances.

***

I play things by ear as I make my way down the South West Coast Path that has now turned into one of those really narrow sea-towny alleys, all the way to the marina. I am enjoying the view of sleepy cats lounging lazily on window ledges and the houseplants left on the front doorsteps of the terraced houses I am walking past. In reality, though, I am battling the desire to just sit in a coffee shop and eat all that there is on display.

I have walked for a while now – probably a couple of hours on the road, then another hour wandering around the town like a lost soul – so I decide to go past Polperro, all the way into the wilderness again, where food isn't available and I can feel a fresh breeze hugging me.

I'm on quite a well-travelled path; lots of dog walkers ascend and descend this stretch of the coastal path daily, just like at Lulworth Cove. I keep going up and down through these vast fields containing nothing but grass and electric fences before I finally come across a stone bench.

I sit and observe how far I've come. Images of golden landscapes and soft clouds are passing by, and I decide this gorgeous spot will do for the night.

***

I am not sure exactly what has changed since I started this journey, but now, when I get lost in my thoughts, they are not all bad ones. Even if it is just for a fraction of a second, sometimes I am able to hold still and find some moments of hope for myself, for my future, that I haven't felt in a while.

Maybe these seven days on the road have shown me that nothing really comes as expected, and that is okay. Maybe what made me feel better was the fact that all of these strangers I encountered along my journey didn't judge me or feel embarrassed around me. Or maybe it is the fact that nature, with its ever-growing and shape-shifting patterns, shows us daily that change is inevitable.

I really don't know why human beings are so obsessed with control and straight lines, but what I do know is that I've really struggled with this fake ideal that everything needs to be planned right down to the details – and that we need to always be happy and in control of our feelings and emotions. It has made me feel as if I'm not good enough to be on this planet.

I've decided that tonight will be my last night out here. Polperro has always been, since I started the walk, just an arbitrary destination that has given me the excuse to keep hiking until I find the meaning of my suffering. I was never really interested in getting to a specific location and although I don't think I've fully grasped what makes my heart ache, what I do know is that I've reached my limit. I think this is the first time that I feel with all of my being that I've had enough of this adventure.

***

At dusk, I set up my bivvy bag, which I've only ended up using once up until now, right at the beginning of the walk. I place it between the sizable rock bench and the path, in the hope that none of my things will tumble down the steep cliff face, and I fall asleep to the whispers of a calming sea. Everything feels as if it's meant to be, and I am very much looking forward to be heading back to Poole tomorrow.

THE LEAP INTO THE PRESENT

The exact moment of the jump into the immensity of the sky,
You realize, anything that comes before and after that,
it is not important whatsoever.
You know that right here right now
is the key for you to just fully embrace it.

And I wonder how many times we forget to do this in life,
Stuck in past moments rethinking what if,
and hoping that the future would bring us what we wish.
But all you need for now,
Is to enjoy the ride and the sound
Of being present.

POOLE:
THE NEW BEGINNING

12 August 2016

The ride home wasn't as straightforward as I thought it would be. I'd kind of forgotten that I had taken several buses and had been on the road for nearly a week non-stop, so obviously I'd covered a considerable distance in this time. In the end, my journey back to Poole involved taking two trains and three buses to make sure I got back the same day.

I can't wait to see the small number of friends I've made during these four months of living in Bournemouth. Most of them are either employees at the climbing centre I go to or random people I bumped into on the beach while I was trying to slackline my days away.

I really love them. They have been an absolute godsend, and have really helped me to get through some tough times. I feel a little guilty because I know how much crap I must have dumped on them to make me feel less shit about myself, and it feels a little unfair, but I hope they understand that I had no other choice.

***

Even though at the start of my summer, I really wanted to try to fill my days with people and commitments, I've learnt that it isn't always possible for me to get everyone's attention all the time. So, I bought myself a pair of climbing shoes and a slackline and I made a vow that these will be my best friends from now on.

I boulder indoors and slackline on the beach, and I'm equally hooked to both. When I slackline, my entire efforts are devoted to placing one foot in front of the other, as I try to balance my entire being on that tight rope. I have fallen down far more times than I have achieved and my legs are constantly covered in bruises, yet I just feel so free. Climbing is my other go-to activity. There's something almost meditative about it, knowing that the only thing I have to do is figure out ways to reach higher. I'm not gonna lie, climbing is absolutely kicking my arse and there are days when I feel super weak and I am so close to giving up, but I don't. Because in that precise moment when I'm throwing my body toward a hold, that hold above me is the only thing in my mind. There isn't me with all my mental health struggles on the wall, there isn't a girl who is about to give up on life. There is just a girl, like many other girls in the world, trying to climb something.

When I climb, just as in life, I am scared, confused, annoyed, angry, tired and committed all at the same time. But, also as in life, if I don't keep going a little further every day, if I am not ripping a layer of skin off several times for the sake of building a thicker one underneath, if I don't stand up and try again after I've lost my grip and fallen clumsily onto the mat... well, if it wasn't for all of that, I would not have made any progress in feeling better and I probably wouldn't even be here today.

My journey to recovery feels like it is never really going to come to an end. Every day I'm learning new things, and sometimes I get very hopeless about it. But then I remember how it feels when I try a climb I can't do yet. It takes focus, strength, coordination, but most of all it takes patience and resilience and those are exactly the same skills I need to stick to my recovery journey. Just like in climbing, I simply have to keep trying until I figure my way to the top, and so I tell myself that maybe it's okay, feeling like I'm never going to stop learning.

The moment I arrive back at my family friend's house, I work up the courage to speak to my host mum about how I have been feeling. Her dog, Ziggy, keeps wagging her tail at me in a show of support, as I explain my situation. Together we decide that seeking professional help is the best course of action. Despite feeling very embarrassed and scared to talk to a professional about how bad things have become, I know deep down this is the right choice for me.

26 August 2016

After a couple of weeks of therapy, I start seeing things around me in a different light. As I sit in Bournemouth Gardens feeding the birds, I am enjoying the taste of freedom that comes with healing from such a consuming mental illness. I am not sitting in fear, avoiding the smell of food or watching enviously as people eat their ice creams. I certainly still feel that same gravitational pull toward eating too much, but I think I am now able to remove the sense of guilt that I was associating with eating tasty things, which was the heaviest and toughest mental process I was having to deal with constantly. I know my inner saboteur is still hiding somewhere, waiting for the first opportunity to jump at me and comment on my body size or my acne. But now, I trust that I have the resilience to just ignore it, or as my therapist says 'inhibit it with kinder words'.

***

I feel incredibly lucky to have met such wonderful people during my first six months of living in England, and although I'm not proud of all my choices in life, I reckon everything that has happened to me so far – even being rejected and mistreated by guys, jobs not going well, and all of the other shitshows I've had to deal with – has at least got me to this exact point in my life. This moment where I feel much more aware of my living body and not so scared to tackle my eating disorder anymore.

Now, at least, I know what it is. Now, thanks to some professional guidance, I know how I can deal with it. I can do it. I can stare at the world with the eyes of a newborn. I can feel the excitement of reliving situations I have experienced thousands of times because they all feel fresh, less heavy, less burdened situations now. I don't always have that chattering voice in my head telling me that I should just disappear from the face of the earth anymore. And that is a huge relief.

***

I open my phone to check my notifications and I realize I have received my admission letter to the International Cultural Arts and Festival Management MA at Manchester Metropolitan University. Wow. I am in! I giggle and chuckle to myself with excitement and decide to cycle home to share the good news. The course starts in only three weeks and I am so excited for this new beginning. It does truly feel like no matter what happens, I will be okay. Now just need to find a place to stay in Manchester!

MANCHESTER:
LIFE IS MESSY, BUT I GOT ME

16 June 2018

It's been a fair while, I know, and I must admit, I lost track of time. I can't believe more than two years have passed since the last time I properly wrote something. But that's just how life flows, right? Some moments seem to be eternal yet some other moments are gone forever before you can even grasp them fully.

But here I am. Alive. Driven again by my gut feeling to bring this diary to completion. For everything and anything that I have experienced, and to put a firm full stop to a journey that feels almost cyclical.

I don't even know where to begin. Life in Manchester has revolutionized a lot of things for me. I moved up north with only the hope of having a new direction, a renewed sense of ambition and drive. I guess what I didn't expect was the impact every single person I encountered up here would have on my life.

I am pleased to say that one of my dreams – to have the full British university experience – came true. As soon as Fresher's Fair hit, I joined the Mountaineering Club and dedicated myself as much as possible to this wonderful bunch of people and the sports we loved so much. I wanted to learn how to climb properly, and this seemed like a good place to start.

Little did I know these people would teach me things way beyond the realm of climbing. Somehow they managed to change my perspective on so many things. I love them all dearly for that. Old Fran went in with the single goal of getting fitter and better at climbing. Present Fran has learnt that there is so much more to the feeling of being physically fit.

I still remember when I first met most of the crew. My eyes were running anxiously over every single person in the room, scrutinizing everyone's weight and physiques. I could sense my mind chatter making nasty comments about whom I deemed overweight. It was a shocking revelation: I – potentially the biggest girl in the room – was desperately trying to find someone fatter than me so I could feel okay about being out socializing, eating and drinking.

***

When I was growing up, being slim meant wearing nice clothes, having a pass to all the coolest parties and social events. Being fat meant having to cover up your body and stay at home so no one would judge you. In Italy, before I left, I barely hung out with anyone who wasn't slim. It wasn't really a conscious choice I made – it never has been the process for me to select friends based on what they look like – but a subconscious act, certainly. Since primary school, I would hear my schoolmates making fun of other people for their size. I have heard kids saying that they don't want to play with them because they're fat. And that was just the start. As I grew up and went to college, I hoped that people would stop focusing so much on people's physical aspects and a little more on their character, but it actually got even worse. I remember specifically there was a very strong and powerful girl, yet a little overweight, in our year at senior school who would do all of the activities that were thought to be reserved for thin, fit people, like pole dancing and burlesque. I can't emphasize enough the insane number of vicious comments that I'd hear my friends make about her weight. She was judged based solely on what she looked like, and not at all for what *she was capable of. I remember I didn't say anything to defend her because I was petrified it would somehow backfire, but also mainly because this 'mean girls attitude was deemed so normal, I wasn't even sure their behaviour was wrong in the first place.*

***

I was 17 then, yet I found myself still stuck in that same loop six years later. And what's worse – I was judging not only others, but myself at the same time. Deeming my own body not worthy of social occasions because of my size, while, in reality, no one around me was bothered about how I looked; they were all just happy I chose to join their club.

One day, it really hit home for me. I was trying to explain to one of my dearest friends how much my eating disorder had changed my body, and then I realized that I was talking about my body as if it was some sort of external, completely disconnected entity I had to deal with. I was calling it my body just for the sake of it, but I may as well have called it 'garbage bin' for the lack of connection I felt with it. I hated it; I wanted to get rid of it, and even when my mental health was getting better, I was struggling to make peace with it.

Soon after this realization I started questioning why so many people, like me, were attached to their physical appearance and thinness as if it were a matter of life or death, and soon realized that those thoughts were never our own thoughts, but rather an ingrained way of thinking that has been spoonfed to us since a young age. The beauty industry keeps reminding people that they're worthless, that they don't deserve a social life, unless they look like the cover model of a magazine. I realized that the guilty feeling that accompanied my overeating was definitely fed by this bullshit idea that fat people are bad people and it made me so angry. I had suffered all these years, hating on my body, thinking I was a monster, only because I grew up in a society that sees diet culture as a solution, instead of as the problem. So, that day, I declared war on diet culture and beauty standards. I promised myself that I was going to start owning my entire body, my physical vessel, the incredible and resilient armature the universe provided me with, and, even more importantly, start taking care of it properly.

What with everything happening in my life – the internal work of accepting my flaws, university assignments, work and climbing – that first year in Manchester flew by. I went from being just okay to being excited about my progress. Then, one day in summer, I was in town, trying to figure out what to bring with me on holiday, when I suddenly felt the overwhelming need to breathe faster, to get out of the crowds. I had been craving a sense of lightness after the hardest year of my life, and instead I felt like there was a crushing weight on my chest. I was having a panic attack. I rushed home to calm my nerves and my breath and got really upset. How could I feel so fine some days and then be back at rock bottom on others?

That afternoon was when I started to get to know her. Miss Anxiety. She's a very subtle lady. She can hide away for months and then, all of sudden, she's right there, in your face. It feels as if no matter what corner of the world you are in, she'll always find you. She will strangle and choke you until you give in. Until you tell yourself that there is nothing you can do to conquer her fully.

Even on brighter days, it's always a battle you've won, never the war. When she appears, she does so fully and ferociously. She keeps you awake, like a monster hiding under the bed. The only way I have been able to deal with her is by pretending I'm fine, because otherwise she just gets to be too much. I pretend I can still fully breathe; I adapt to the way the breath becomes shallower and my heartbeat races. It's adaptation, not survival; it's surrender, not victory. At first, I thought she was triggered by people and situations, so I removed myself from as many uncomfortable settings as I could. But then, I realized Miss Anxiety was mainly created in my head, and the only way to find relief from her was either suffocating her with tons of food, or let her burst into a panic attack.

That was when I truly tapped into how hard recovery was going to be. In my naïve mind, I pictured this utopic version of events, where I would admit to suffer with mental health issues and then I would be feeling okay again.

If only that were true.

Unfortunately, this whole process of regaining ownership of my own thoughts wasn't so simple. Recovering from an eating disorder takes a lot of mental strength. Everything I used to do, everything I used to think, every little habit I had – it all needed to be re-calibrated. My actions, once driven by the concept of perfectionism and self-hate, needed to become gestures of love and kindness toward myself. The thought of not being good enough needed to be forcefully (at first) replaced with 'I am okay.' Every time I caught myself examining every little imperfection of my body, I needed to change that action into one of gentle caressing and acceptance.

I didn't always like it. It still feels sometimes like I'm lying to myself when I try to repeat, 'I love my body' or 'I am enough'.

It felt scary and overwhelming – like an effort that will last a lifetime. Especially since my brain had been starved of self-compassion for such a long time, planting the one and only seed of self-respect seems pointless.

However, after writing, reflecting and (over-)analysing, I realized that that was probably the closest to being human I've ever gotten: creating a healthy image of myself and taking care of it.

It had been nearly a year and a half since I'd broken up with my ex, and I remember wanting someone by my side so desperately. I missed that incredible feeling of releasing all of my sorrows and demons into the arms of someone I loved, and who loved me.

Sure, it would have been nice to meet someone and spend some time together, but I was actually really fed up with all of the pressure that us girls and women have to go through just to be liked. Honestly, it's a joke! All I hear is this ongoing commentary on how girls are either too much or not enough; too hard to get, too easy to sleep with; too straightforward, too flirty, too easy-going, too strong, too smiley, too loud, too chatty, too masculine, too sincere... The list goes on and on. I couldn't begin to count the number of times I've been told I should have tried to be nicer, cooler, more desirable. What am I? A thing? A new toy? According to society, women always seem to have to change something about themselves in order to deserve an external source of love, affection and security.

That was when it all started making sense. Piece by piece, I had been annihilating my soul for the likes of other people I didn't even need. I denied little chunks of myself – my dreams, hopes and expectations – until I denied my whole being. And what have I gained from this? Nothing but a huge bag of self-hate, body dysmorphia, mental health issues, dependence on other people's judgements – oh, and let's not forget an eating disorder. I was so through with it.

So, I made a vow. A vow to myself that for every word of self-hatred and negative self-talk I subjected myself to, I had to say or do five nice things for myself.

This has unarguably been the most important change I've made in my recovery. To promise to stand up for myself and dedicate all of the love songs and cheesy romantic gestures to me, myself and I. I didn't need an external reason or a boyfriend to feel loved.

Funnily enough, a couple of months after I realized that I shouldn't have given a single fuck about what other people thought of me, a very attractive, energetic and assertive guy came into my life. It was nice to finally date someone who wasn't so attached to just my physical aspect and aesthetics, but liked everything about me.

The late 2017, early 2018 years for me were very transitional. I had just finished all of my uni assignments and was meant to be handing in my dissertation. I know part of me was super excited about accomplishing a 2:1 master's degree in a second language, but somehow I managed to get super anxious about it all. I believe a part of me didn't want the uni experience to end.

I started exercising mindfully again, after a sequence of terrible failed attempts at joining local gyms, thanks to a movement coach that went above and beyond the physical realms of the body, and introduced me to powerful tools like meditation and breathing techniques. Skoti, his name, Fera, his company name, stepped into my life that year as the guide that reminded me, every step of the way, that change was possible only when I started believing in it.

My tenancy contract was also expiring so I decided to move in with my closest friend from the Mountaineering Club, and we spent the days watching *RuPaul's Drag Race* and going out in the park slacklining. We really bonded, confessing to each other all our deepest hurts, and we would laugh, cry and support each other because, to us, that was the only way out of our misery. So, I was very thankful I'd found someone who understood me without needing to speak. It made my life a little easier and a little more bearable. I had gone nearly a full month without having a binge-eating episode and I started being able to look at my body and find it somewhat attractive. I was able, for the first time in years, to wear lingerie or swimming suits without hating every inch of my skin or wishing my fat away.

While I was slowly and carefully making my way out of six years of self-hate and destruction, I began to also realize that my best friend was only just starting her journey of self acceptance and emotional healing. There was a lot that I wanted to tell her, do for her, but I was so unsure how to even begin. On top of that, she didn't feel comfortable around the person I started seeing romantically due to her own recent break-up, so I was finding myself split between the two of them, my dearest friend and my partner. I felt torn; I needed to protect my own newly re-acquired energy, but at the same time I wanted to at least try to dig her out of her misery like we used to for each other just the year before. It was very painful. I really hated myself for doing what I did afterwards, but I am aware now that it was really the only move I could have made. As hard as it was, my mental health had to take priority, so I stepped away. I tapped out. At the end of the tenancy I moved out, with the guy I was in a relationship with.

I felt so guilty about it at first, it felt like I was stabbing in the back the only person who has ever understood and felt my pain, but I now know it wasn't in my power to save her from herself. She needed to learn to do that on her own, just like I had to do for myself, because I wasn't going to be there forever and I could not have substituted professional help.

This may seem really cruel to say, but for me, it was another major breakthrough in my recovery journey.

The simplest and scariest of all truths needed to be heard and learnt time after time, as I was stuck in a loop of feeling like a victim of anything that happened or didn't happen to me. I felt powerless for a very long time, as if people around me were the only ones able to influence my own life, for better or for worse. As if I could have just relied on that special someone that was going to arrive and save me from myself. The hard truth is that the only person that will always be with me, for the rest of my life – unconditionally and sometimes a little unwillingly – is me. And when I really grasped that concept of knowing that my own company would be my only guaranteed company from the start to the end of my life, that's when I decided I needed to make it a good one. No more acting like I wasn't in charge of my own destiny. From that moment on, I was going to be the support I was always looking for in others. I was going to learn how to be a better ally to myself.

***

MY HOME

So grateful.
For the past
Has taught me
A lesson never to be forgotten
the meaning of H O M E
Body and town.
As this is where I'm from
No other place to feel at ease.
It is funny how I have tried to cease
Several times the relationship, the life
I had built in between.
Tried to deny
Or forget
The powerful connection
I was made of
Making me wanna get rid
Of them all.
But like body, like town,
This is my temple,
My ground
And every time I come back
After being away,
It makes me appreciate
Twice as much when I stay.
Blissfully hard lesson,
I will constantly keep learning.

***

01 February 2019

It's now been nearly a year and half since I had any major episodes of bingeing. After that eye-opening moment of realization where I realized I needed to be an ally to myself, life got even busier with 'adult' stuff and people I cared about. I seemed to have completely disconnected from my need to write, yet these words became my 'must re-read' any time I was feeling wobbly about my recovery from binge-eating and related catastrophes. I remember the first time I was able to leave something on my plate because my body was actually communicating clearly to my brain that I was full. That was such a milestone for me that I rang my mum in tears to tell her how good it felt. I also remember, though, that I had to fight off the other voice in my head telling me I should be ashamed for leaving food on the plate while so many around the world were starving. My eating disorder was giving me guilt for my 'first-world problem' and not eating all of what I had been offered. After that, my brain also tried to replace the lack of comfort foods with tonnes of panic attacks, but at that point, going to therapy had become so much less stressful that I really delved deeper into my feelings and started figuring out the whys and the hows of my anxiety.

As much as I would love to write a formula on how to get myself out of a future encounter with my eating disorder, I can't.

Firstly, I don't think it ended at all. I am just much more aware now of it happening and it allows me, most of the time, to have that extra minute to reflect before I act irrationally and start going down the road of self-hatred and starvation again. If there is one thing that really helped me to not feel defeated or lost completely when facing another episode, it was all the facts I had learned about eating disorders.

I remember one day, I went all out and borrowed five books from the library just to learn more about the common causes, triggers and subsequent behaviours of those who suffer from eating disorders, so that I could be alert to them when it was happening to me. That was very helpful, but, alas, often knowing about a problem is not enough. For me, it was really hard to break old and dangerous patterns because I had been stuck with them for so long that my brain just didn't know any better.

I realized I was basically dealing with a needy inner child. My conscious and adult brain had to reteach everything I knew to my suffering inner child so that I could learn to swap hurtful habits and ways of thinking with more useful ones. Among other things, I had to reteach myself how to take care of myself, how to cook for myself, how to eat in front of people, how to cope with buffets, and more. I also had to relearn how to understand whether or not I was really hungry or if my hunger was a symptom of something else, like tiredness, or nervousness, or an emotional response to something that was bothering me. Hardest of all, however, I had to first learn how to re-appreciate all types of foods, without feeling guilty.

***

RESET

I like letting go
of educational preconceptions
Learning
how to deal with the world
In my own way and not the way my mum told me.
She is she
I am me.
And she sees
A fire
Never burnt in herself
Something she couldn't tell
What is made of and
Where it stems
But I know,
This fire burns
Because I scratched my skin
To create kindle
And adventure is my spark.

Always ready to depart
I am burning strongly in the wind
of change.

***

For seven years, food controlled my thoughts daily, to the point that I can't recall a single moment where I really tasted or enjoyed what I was eating. I saw food either as the only way out of my problems or the only problem I'd ever had. For nearly seven years of my life, society had pushed and shoved into my brain the idea that there are bad foods and good foods, and that I am, accordingly, a good or bad person depending on what I choose to eat. Not only did I have to burn that idea down and bury it deep under the ground, I also had to dismantle the notion that my worth was defined by what size jeans I wore. I had to relearn how to exercise without punishing myself, coming away from the mentality of 'no pain, no gain', and, most of all, from counting how many calories I had burnt versus how many calories I had eaten. I literally threw away my scales; I just don't need that number in my life anymore.

I was angry at society, and I still am, for the ridiculous and severely lacking education we receive about mental health. One day, though, I tapped into that repressed anger and disgust I had for the complete normalization of body dysmorphia and disordered eating patterns that our society displays, and I had another major breakthrough. That anger I was feeling inside, raging and burning, was transforming into such fierce power that pushed me through my toughest days, I can't even begin to describe it. My suffering was giving me the will to be brave and endure it all, just so I could come out the other side and lend a hand to anyone who was utterly lost and broken by it. So that no one else I could reach would suffer in silence about this.

UNCONDITIONALLY ME

I am not gonna lie,
I will probably change my mind a thousand times.
But the way forward,
That, to me
Only exists outside the box.
And how do I know what's outside
If I even never really got up and tried?

I'm not gonna lie
I do love my life.
It's not about the money I make or
the risk that I take
It's always about connections
And reflections
Under a clear sky

I couldn't live any other way
It makes me sick thinking I would be swayed
For different a cause
Rather than the human flaws
I make weird choices
But my voices
Are telling me to follow though
So that's me.

***

I guess what I am trying to say is that the struggle is still real,
but at least I now know what the struggle entails, instead of
fumbling around in the dark, completely unaware of it all.

All in all, I now look at that demon, that shadow I carried around secretively for so many years, and I am grateful for the roller coaster I was given. Sure, I would have preferred not to suffer so much as a result of my body image, but, equally, that suffering has given me so much strength. When things with that guy I was dating didn't go as planned, I cried, I shouted, and I was very sad – but I wasn't *broken*. I wasn't *lost*. I didn't get to a point where I didn't know who I was anymore. And that, to me, meant more than anything on the planet.

I was so relieved (and I'll admit, also a little surprised) that I was able to hold on to my integrity, my sense of self, and overcome this setback in true Fran style. I packed my bags, quit my boring job, moved my belongings, and slept on friends' couches until the day I flew to India to complete my Yoga Teacher Training Course. A dream was coming true, and it was growing from the very mud I had found myself in when breaking up with that guy. Old Fran would have defined herself as someone's girlfriend and felt utterly bereft. New Fran was okay.

***

GROWING PAINS

Stitching my heart
Shouldn't be so hard
After multiple tries

I wonder what it takes
To restart again
Without fearing the possibility
Of having to micro
Fracture the integrity
Of my soul
And the unlimited power

Of my love
again
Oh wait
That's it
I know now
There's no remedy
To the pain
You get from the truth
But it's the purest
And most liberating
Chance
Of growth

So let it be
The reality
Can come at me
And caress my face
Or bring me down
Depending on what I need
And what the universe
Sees
Yet unknown to me.

***

New Fran held on to herself like never before, because she was certain that nothing was ever going to be as hard or as difficult as having to fight against her own mind. Against all of those self-destructive thoughts she had been hearing in her head for such a long time. New Fran knew she was going to be okay. She knew that she was going to figure everything out, just like she had done before.

***

INDIA

Last minute decisions,
Contrasting opinions,
My head telling me to be rational and my heart imploring me
to open my eyes.
Friends who went mad
Few things to unpack

From my eight boxes of Mancunian life, all to fit into a bright
yellow duffel bag
The emotional roller coaster of applying
Not knowing if the visa would be a fake
The flight would not be too late
The choice would just not be the right choice.
Quitting work in a rush,
Compress my feelings into stacks
of books and knowledge I need to ingest before the
departure.
5 couches, 2 bags, 2 flights, one cold sore and a lot of never
ending day time

All to be here,
in awe of this fear
That all of a sudden has transformed in hope
And joy
The sadness replaced by that thrilling sense of the
unexplored unknown
and all the possible futures
that I opened up today,
by saying YAY!
To the powerful and blind desire of self love and self care and
self development.

Life is tough.
And messy.
And full of surprises.
A little bit like India itself.

EPILOGUE

28 May 2020

Dear diary,

Something quite unexpected happened when I was travelling and visiting marvellous places.

I am not sure why, nor how, but I once again became extremely body-aware.

I started pinching my fat rolls like I used to do when I first wrote these pages. I started panicking about how much I would be eating while doing so little exercise, and I really struggled with my body image in reflective surfaces like mirrors and windows. My body dysmorphia was making me wear baggy and long clothing in order to cover up any flaws.

However, rather than feeling scary, this time it felt incredibly exhausting. Going through each stage of a relapse, having not felt this way for so long, really lowered my self-esteem, yet it didn't feel like an unknown situation – more like I was about to repeat school from scratch. I could see myself reliving the same ups and downs, the same draining hours spent in front of the mirror retraining my brain that fat doesn't necessarily mean unhealthy and that cellulite isn't a death sentence.

After all of these insane battles against my own thought patterns, I came to realize that maybe becoming bigger as a person isn't so bad after all.

I can't expect my body to remain the exact same way it was when I was 15. I need to accept the fact that, as a grown woman, I hold more experience, more life, more memories in this body than I have ever done before. That's a beautiful thing, so why do I look at my bigger body and consider myself unworthy of love, attention and care?

***

SHRINKING ISN'T FOR ME

You want to know the truth?
I am human too.
You want to keep it real?
The feelings ain't always so good.
And in this pursuit of purpose and happiness
I tend to forget that my body is my vehicle
I grow to make space for more knowledge and passion,
I expand when my limitations shrink.

Reducing my value to a size is
NOT a process of growth,
if anything it is the annihilation of my soul.
I do not want that.
I want to be one with nature,
I want to be a genuine
Caring
Loving creature.

***

If there is one thing I have learnt on this never-ending journey of battling my eating disorder, it is that the more I wish for this to end, the more painful I am going to make it for myself. For me, it has always come down to finding unrelated internal and external reasons to start getting better.

That's probably why the period after I got back to Manchester from India seemed to slip through my hands. I started dating again; I found a job and a house. I rebuilt my life from the foundations of my new soul and it felt really good. I had been hustling and running around to make my yoga classes thrive with no time to stop whatsoever. After only three months of running classes, I saw the opportunity to make it a full-time job and I didn't think twice. That, right there, for me, was the exact drive I needed to invest more time and energy into what I loved and less time and energy in my self-destructive mind chatter.

My reasons to recover, my reasons to stay alive, have substituted the pain I was carrying inside for so many years with ambition, passion and a little nudge of confidence.

And then March 2020 arrived, and the world stopped. Not the animals running, not the plants growing, not the Earth looping around the sun, but all of humanity had to be put on pause.

I knew, from the first few weeks, that this new way of life was going to be very challenging. Being sat at home, without much of an income, with that much time on my hands and not a lot of things to distract my brain, sounded extremely dangerous in my journey to complete recovery.

Yet I also knew that just because it was challenging, it didn't have to mean I couldn't overcome it.

I don't think I have ever dedicated so much time to myself. I slept for all those times I couldn't sleep as a child, I read all of the books that had sat unread on my wish list for ages, I revised some Mandarin and other interesting things I had learned at uni, I sat in the sun and pretended I was in Italy again and when I felt strong enough, I tried to sit with all of the feelings that I have ever felt, especially those uncomfortable ones that make me think horrible things about myself. I sat, and as they surfaced, I wrote them all down. And then I cried.

I cried for days. I cried openly about all of the hurt I have experienced and also all of the hurt that I may have caused to other people. And it felt good. It felt like I had finally found my closure. I was finally at peace with myself, trusting that I was going to deal with everything else in my life going forward just as I learnt from my adventure on the South West Coast Path – one step at a time.

***

LOCKDOWN GRACE

Here I lie
Suspended in time
Making myself one with the rhythm of the earth
Discovering
treasures in
Slow motion

Freedom through sensation

My body is rooting, stilling, growing.
My mind is awakening, redefining, accepting.
It never felt so good before
learning how to forgive myself.

ACKNOWLEDGEMENTS

I would like to thank quite a few people for the support I received whilst bringing this project to life.

Firstly, my dear friend Virginia, who was the first person I spoke to about my mental health struggles. She listened to me and helped me to realize that there are so many people out there every day who are silently facing the same issues.

Secondly, I would like to thank my family for allowing me to have some space and distance when I needed to work on myself, and for always trusting my approach to recovery without interfering.

Thirdly, Emma Salazar, who sat patiently listening to my project and helped me to create the story I share in this book.

Finally, I want to acknowledge and thank everyone who has been there since my first mental health blog was born: my climbing crew in Manchester, who supported me through some of my most difficult times, Grant Langton, for being such a cool human and creating the most beautiful illustration for the front cover, and my partner Leon Wilson, for believing in me when I struggle to do so.

ABOUT CHERISH EDITIONS

Cherish Editions is a bespoke self-publishing service for authors of mental health, wellbeing and inspirational books.

As a division of Trigger Publishing, the UK's leading independent mental health and wellbeing publisher, we are experienced in creating and selling positive, responsible, important and inspirational books, which work to de-stigmatize the issues around mental health and improve the mental health and wellbeing of those who read our titles.

Founded by Adam Shaw, a mental health advocate, author and philanthropist, and leading psychologist Lauren Callaghan, Cherish Editions aims to publish books that provide advice, support and inspiration. We nurture our authors so that their stories can unfurl on the page, helping them to share their uplifting and moving stories.

Cherish Editions is unique in that a percentage of the profits from the sale of our books goes directly to leading mental health charity Shawmind, to deliver its vision to provide support for those experiencing mental ill health.

Find out more about Cherish Editions by visiting cherisheditions.com or by joining us on:
Twitter @cherisheditions
Facebook @cherisheditions
Instagram @cherisheditions

Cherish
EDITIONS

ABOUT SHAWMIND

A proportion of profits from the sale of all Trigger books go to their sister charity, Shawmind, also founded by Adam Shaw and Lauren Callaghan. The charity aims to ensure that everyone has access to mental health resources whenever they need them.

You can find out more about the work Shawmind do by visiting their website: shawmind.org or joining them on:

Twitter @Shaw_Mind
Facebook @ShawmindUK
Instagram @Shaw_Mind

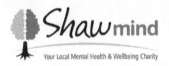

Lightning Source UK Ltd.
Milton Keynes UK
UKHW040658100821
388619UK00001B/38